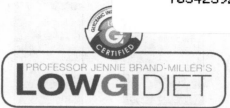

Make healthy carb choices easy with the
Shopper's Guide

OTHER TITLES IN THE **LOW GI DIET** SERIES

GI BASICS

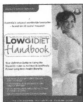

WEIGHT-LOSS

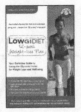

COOKBOOKS

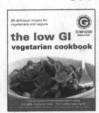
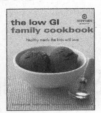

DIABETES AND PRE-DIABETES

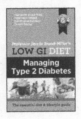

COELIAC DISEASE
OR GLUTEN
INTOLERANCE

FERTILITY AND PCOS

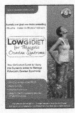
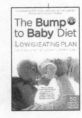
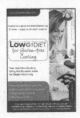

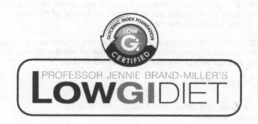

PROFESSOR JENNIE BRAND-MILLER'S
LOWGIDIET

Make healthy carb choices easy with the
Shopper's Guide

Now includes gluten-free foods

PROF JENNIE BRAND-MILLER
KAYE FOSTER-POWELL
DR FIONA ATKINSON

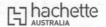
hachette
AUSTRALIA

hachette
AUSTRALIA

First published in Australia and New Zealand in 2005
by Hodder Australia
(An imprint of Hachette Australia Pty Limited)
Level 17, 207 Kent Street, Sydney NSW 2000
www.hachette.com.au

Revised editions published by Hachette Australia in 2006, 2007, 2008, 2009, 2010, 2011, 2012, 2013, 2014, 2015
This revised edition published in 2016

National Library of Australia Cataloguing-in-Publication data:

Brand Miller, Janette, 1952– author.
Low GI diet shopper's guide / Prof Jennie Brand-Miller;
Kaye Foster-Powell; Dr Fiona Atkinson.

978 0 7336 3548 9 (pbk.)

Glycemic index.
Food – carbohydrate content.
Diet therapy.
Foster-Powell, Kaye, author.
Atkinson, Fiona, author.

613.283

Front cover images: Shutterstock (shopping bag and groceries); iStockPhoto (potatoes and pasta)
Cover design by Seymour Designs
Original text design by Pindar NZ, Auckland, New Zealand
Tables adaptation by Kirby Jones
Printed and bound in Australia by McPherson's Printing Group

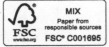

Contents

10 steps to a healthy low GI life for everybody, every day, every meal

- ❏ Eat seven or more servings of fruit and vegetables every day
- ❏ Eat low GI breads and cereals, especially wholegrain versions
- ❏ Eat more legumes including soybeans, chickpeas and lentils
- ❏ Eat small portions of nuts every day
- ❏ Eat more fish and seafood
- ❏ Eat lean red meat, poultry and eggs
- ❏ Eat low fat dairy foods or calcium-enriched soy products
- ❏ Eat less saturated fat and replace with good mono- and poly-unsaturated fats
- ❏ Moderate your alcohol intake and use of salt
- ❏ Be active – don't sit for long periods. Even 30 seconds of activity will rev up your metabolism

Understanding
the GI

Using the *Shopper's Guide*

We have put together this handy guide full of GI values to help you put those low GI smart carb food choices into your shopping trolley and onto your plate. By doing so, you'll satisfy your hunger, increase your energy levels, and eliminate your desire to eat more than you should.

Some foods that have been tested by accredited laboratories display the certified GI symbol. But what about the rest? With tables listing the GI of hundreds of foods – from breads and breakfast bars to fruit juice, fruit and vegetables – this book will save you time in the supermarket by directing you to the best low GI foods available.

You can use the GI tables on pages 99–197 to:

❏ Find the GI of your favourite foods

❏ Compare foods within a category (two types of bread for example)

❏ Improve your diet by finding a low GI substitute for high GI foods

❏ Put together a low GI meal

❏ Shop for low GI foods.

What are the benefits of low GI carbs?

Knowing the GI values of individual foods is your key to the enormous health benefits of a low GI diet.

Low GI eating has science on its side. It's not a 'diet' in the popular sense. There are no strict rules or regimens to follow. It's essentially about making simple adjustments to your usual eating habits – such as swapping one type of bread or breakfast cereal for another.

You'll find that you can live with it for life.

Low GI eating:

❏ Reduces swings in blood glucose
❏ Reduces your insulin levels and helps you burn fat
❏ Lowers your cholesterol levels
❏ Helps control your appetite
❏ Reduces your risk of heart disease and diabetes
❏ Is suitable for your whole family
❏ Means you are eating foods closer to the way nature intended
❏ Doesn't defy commonsense!

Not only that. You will feel better and have more energy – and you don't have to deprive or discipline yourself. A low GI diet is easy and has particular benefits for people who are overweight, have diabetes, hypertension, elevated blood fats, heart disease or the metabolic syndrome (Syndrome X).

Understanding the GI of foods helps you choose the right amount of carbohydrate and the right sort of carbohydrate for your longterm health and wellbeing.

The GI explained

The GI is a physiologically based measure of the effect of carbohydrates on blood glucose levels. It provides an easy and delicious way to eat a healthy diet and at the same time control fluctuations in blood glucose. After testing hundreds of foods around the world, scientists have found that mixed meals with a low GI will have less of an effect on blood glucose levels than those with a high GI.

❑ Carbohydrates that break down rapidly during digestion, releasing glucose quickly into the bloodstream have a high GI.

❑ Carbohydrates that break down slowly, releasing glucose gradually into the bloodstream, have a low GI.

The rate of carbohydrate digestion has important implications for everybody. For most people, foods with a low GI have advantages over those with a high GI. They can:

❑ Improve blood glucose control

❑ Increase satiety as they are more filling and satisfying and reduce appetite

❑ Facilitate weight loss

❑ Improve blood fat profiles

❑ Reduce risk of developing type 2 diabetes, heart disease and certain types of cancer.

A low GI diet helps people:

❑ With type 1 diabetes

❑ With type 2 diabetes

- ❏ With pre-diabetes (who may have been told they have 'a touch of diabetes' or impaired glucose tolerance)
- ❏ With gestational diabetes (diabetes during pregnancy)
- ❏ With hypoglycemia or low blood glucose
- ❏ With insulin resistance or high insulin levels
- ❏ Who are overweight or obese
- ❏ Who have lost weight and want to prevent weight re-gain
- ❏ Who are at a normal weight but have too much fat around the middle (abdominal overweight)
- ❏ With higher than desirable blood glucose levels
- ❏ With high levels of triglycerides
- ❏ With low levels of HDL cholesterol ('good' cholesterol)
- ❏ With metabolic syndrome
- ❏ With polycystic ovarian syndrome (PCOS) (irregular periods, acne, facial hair)
- ❏ With non-alcoholic fatty liver (NAFL) disease or non-alcoholic steatohepatitis (NASH)
- ❏ Who want to delay or prevent age-related vision problems
- ❏ Who want to prevent all of the above and live a long and healthy life.

If you would like to know more about the beneficial effects eating low GI foods can have on the above conditions, please refer to our other books – a full list is shown at the beginning of this guide.

About the authors

Professor Jennie Brand-Miller is an internationally recognised authority on carbohydrates and health. She is Professor of Human Nutrition at the University of Sydney and a past Chair of the National Nutrition Committee of the Australian Academy of Science.

Kaye Foster-Powell is an accredited practising dietitian with extensive experience in diabetes management and a longstanding interest in the practical application of the glycemic index.

Dr Fiona Atkinson is a research dietitian and the manager of the Sydney University Glycemic Index Research Service (SUGiRS). Her research focuses on investigating the genetic and lifestyle factors that influence carbohydrate digestion and glucose metabolism.

We would like to thank the dedicated GI testing team at SUGiRS – Courtney Wright, Clair de Sousa, Alisha Li, Stephanie Yong and Reece Adler – and all our cheerful, well-fed and patient volunteers. We would also like to thank Associate Professor Gareth Denyer for his invaluable help with the GI database and Dr Alan Barclay from the GI Symbol Program for the sugars and sweeteners information and for thoroughly checking the GI tables for us. Thank you to dietitian Dr Kate Marsh who helped us with the gluten-free section on pages 65–72, *GI News* editor Philippa Sandall and everyone at Hachette Australia who has worked so hard on our behalf, especially Fiona Hazard, Karen Ward and Nathan Grice.

Low GI
eating

3 steps to a balanced low GI meal

1 is for carb

It's an essential, although sometimes maligned, part of a balanced meal. What do you feel like? A grain like rice, barley or cracked wheat? Pasta, noodles or bean vermicelli? Or perhaps a high carb vegetable like sweet corn, sweet potato or legumes? Include at least one low GI carb per meal.

2 is for protein

Include some protein at each meal. It lowers the glycemic load by replacing *some* of the carbohydrate – not all! It also helps satisfy the appetite.

3 is for fruit and vegetables

This is the part we often go without. If anything it should have the highest priority in a meal, but a meal based solely on fruit and low carb vegetables won't be sustaining for long. A plain salad sandwich is a recipe for hunger.

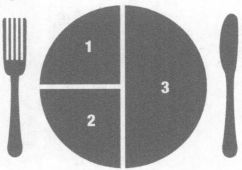

Making the change

Eating the low GI way simply involves replacing high GI foods in your diet with low GI foods. This could mean eating muesli at breakfast instead of wheat flakes, low GI bread instead of normal white or wholemeal bread, or a sparkling apple juice in place of a soft drink.

You don't need to count numbers or do any sort of mental arithmetic to make sure you are eating a healthy low GI diet.

Tips for putting the GI into practice

Be aware! Only carbohydrate-containing foods have GI values

The diet we eat contains three main nutrients: protein, carbohydrate and fat. Some foods, such as meat, are high in protein, while bread is high in carbohydrate and butter is high in fat. We need to consume a variety of foods (in varying proportions) to provide all three nutrients, but the GI applies only to carbohydrate-rich foods. It is impossible for us to measure a GI value for foods like meat which contain negligible carbohydrate. The same applies to cheese, egg, avocado, butter, oil and alcohol. It is incorrect to refer to these foods as high or low GI. There are other nutritional aspects which you should consider when choosing these foods: for example, the amount and type of fats they contain.

The GI is not intended to stand alone

We don't categorise foods as 'good' or 'bad' according to their GI. While you will benefit from eating low GI foods at each meal, this doesn't have to be at the exclusion of all others. High GI foods like most potatoes and bread still make valuable nutritional contributions to our diet. And low GI foods like pastry that are high in saturated fat are no better for us because of their low GI. The nutritional benefits of different foods are many and varied, and it is advisable for you to base your food choices on the overall nutritional content of a food, particularly considering the saturated fat, salt and fibre in addition to GI.

You don't need to add up the GI each day

In some of our early books we included sample menus and calculated an estimated GI for the day. As our understanding of the GI grew and we talked to our clients and heard from our readers, we realised this made life complicated for them. No calculations are necessary! Although we can predict the GI of a menu for the whole day, we can't predict the GI of many recipes, especially those using flour. That's why we now prefer simply to categorise foods as low, medium or high GI in most circumstances. We have also found that many people who substitute high with low GI foods in their everyday meals and snacks reduce the overall GI of their diet, gain better blood glucose control and lose weight.

You don't need to be pedantic about GI values

Whether a food's GI is 59 or 61 isn't biologically relevant. Normal day-to-day variation in the human body could obscure the difference in these values.

This for that – substituting high GI with low GI foods

Simply substituting high GI foods with low GI alternatives will give your overall diet a lower GI and deliver the benefits of low GI eating. Here's how you can put slow carbs to work by cutting back high GI foods and replacing them with alternatives that are just as tasty.

If you are currently eating this (high GI) food	Choose this (low GI) alternative instead
Biscuits	A slice of wholegrain bread or toast with jam or fruit spread
Breads such as soft white or wholemeal; smooth textured breads, rolls, scones, dampers	Dense breads with wholegrains, wholegrain and stoneground flour and sourdough. Look for the low GI symbol
Breakfast cereals – most commercial, processed cereals including cornflakes, Rice Bubbles, cereal 'biscuits'	Traditional rolled oats, muesli and the commercial low GI brands listed in the tables. Look for the low GI symbol
Cakes and pastries	Raisin toast, fruit loaf and fruit buns are healthier baked options; yoghurts and low fat mousses also make great snacks or desserts
Chips and other packet snacks such as Twisties, pretzels, Burger Rings	Fresh fruit, nuts and trail mix

If you are currently eating this (high GI) food	Choose this (low GI) alternative instead
Crackers	Crisp vegetable strips such as carrot, capsicum or celery
Hot chips and French fries	Leave them out! Have salad or extra vegetables instead. Corn on the cob or coleslaw are better takeaway options
Lollies	Chocolate is lower GI but high in fat. Healthier options are sultanas, dried apricots and other dried fruit
Muesli bars	Try a nut bar or dried fruit and nut mix.
Potatoes	Look for Australia's only low GI potato – Carisma – on supermarket shelves. You can also try sweet potato, yam, taro or baby new potatoes – or just replace with other low GI or no-GI vegetables
Rice, especially large servings of it in dishes such as risotto, nasi goreng, fried rice	Try Basmati or SunRice Doongara low GI Clever rice or low GI brown rice, pearled barley, cracked wheat (bulgur), quinoa, pasta or noodles. Look for the low GI symbol
Soft drink and fruit juice	Use a diet variety if you drink these often. Fruit juice has a lower GI (but it is not a lower kilojoule option). Water or milk is best
Sugar	Moderate the quantity. Consider pure wildflower honey, apple juice, LoGiCane, fructose (such as Fruisana) and grape nectar as alternatives. Look for the low GI symbol

Your GI Q&A

Does low carb automatically mean low GI?

Not at all. Low carb is *just about quantity*; it simply means that a food or meal does not contain much carbohydrate. It says nothing about the quality of the carbs in the food or meal on your plate. You could be eating a low carb meal but the carbs have a medium or high GI. Low GI on the other hand is *all about quality*. Whether you are a moderate or high carb eater, low GI carbs (dense wholegrain breads, legumes/pulses, many fruits and vegetables) will have significant health benefits – promoting weight control, reducing your blood glucose and insulin levels throughout the day, and increasing your sense of feeling full and satisfied after eating. We suggest that you make the most of quality carbs and reap the add-on health benefits such as:

❏ vitamin E from wholegrain cereals

❏ vitamin C, beta-carotene and potassium from fruits and vegetables

❏ vitamin B6 from bananas and wholegrain cereals

❏ pantothenic acid, zinc, iron and magnesium from wholegrains and legumes

❏ anti-oxidants and phytochemicals from all plant foods

❏ and fibre which comes from all of the above and doesn't come from any animal food.

Why do many high-fibre foods have a high GI value?
Dietary fibre is not one chemical constituent like fat and protein. It is composed of many different sorts of molecules and can be divided into soluble and insoluble types. Soluble fibre is often viscous (thick and jelly-like) in solution and remains viscous even in the small intestine. For this reason it makes it harder for enzymes to move around and digest the food. Foods with more-soluble fibre, like apples, oats, and legumes, therefore have low GI values.

Insoluble fibre, on the other hand, is not viscous and doesn't slow digestion unless it's acting like a fence to inhibit access by enzymes (e.g. the bran around intact kernels). When insoluble fibre is finely milled, the enzymes have free reign, allowing rapid digestion. Wholemeal bread and white bread have similar GI values. Brown pasta and brown rice have similar values to their white counterparts.

Should I avoid all high GI foods?
There is no need to eat only low GI foods. While you will benefit from eating low GI foods at each meal, this doesn't have to be at the exclusion of all others. When eaten with protein foods or low GI foods, the overall GI value of the meal will be about medium.

What GI number should a person aim for when trying to diet?

The simple answer is there's no formula. You don't need to add up the GI each day. In fact there's no counting at all as there is with calories/kilojoules. The basic technique for eating the low GI way is simply swapping the high GI carbs in your diet with low GI foods. So, what you need to aim for is identifying the high GI carbs in your current diet and swapping them for nutritious sources of low GI carbs. When you're looking at GI values, it's best to compare like with like – one bread with another, for example – rather than 'bread' with 'fruit'. This way you'll be comparing foods of similar nutritional value, which will help you to make an appropriate swap from the high GI to the low GI version. Try keeping the simple guidelines on page 16 in mind.

Guidelines

Every day:

❑ Eat at least three meals – don't skip meals. Eat snacks too if you are hungry.

❑ Eat fruit at least twice – fresh, cooked, dried, juices.

❑ Eat vegetables at least twice – cooked, raw, salads, soups, juices and snacks.

❑ Eat a cereal at least once – bread, breakfast cereal, pasta, noodles, rice and other grains in a wholegrain or low GI form.

❑ Accumulate 60 minutes of physical activity (including incidental activity and planned exercise).

Every week:

❑ Eat beans, peas and/or lentils – at least twice. This includes baked beans, chickpeas, red kidney beans, butter beans, split peas and foods made from them such as hommus and dhal.

❑ Eat fish and seafood at least once, preferably three times – fresh, smoked, frozen or canned.

❑ Eat nuts most days – just a small handful.

Low GI
shopping

Planning to shop

The perfect place to get started on healthy low GI eating is the supermarket, whether you are pushing a trolley up and down the aisles, or shopping online. This is where we make those hurried or impulsive decisions that have a big impact.

Spend a little time each day, or weekly if it suits, planning what to eat when. It makes life simpler. Meal planning is just writing down what you intend to eat for the main meals of the week, then checking your fridge and pantry for ingredients available and noting what you need to purchase.

Our shopping list on pages 22–33 will help you stock the pantry and fridge with the staples you require to turn out a meal in minutes. To make your own shopping list, use the same headings. They will take you to the appropriate aisles of the supermarket or to the shops you usually favour. We've included convenience foods such as canned beans, bagged salads, ready-made hummus, bottled sauces and pastes, canned fruits and chopped vegetables (fresh and frozen) but you may prefer to make your own if you have time.

Making sense of food labelling

Often we're asked questions like: 'What should I look for on the label?' and 'Can I believe what it says?' There's a lot of information on food labels these days, but unfortunately, very few people know how to interpret it correctly. Often the claims on the front of the packet don't quite mean what you think.

Here are some prime examples:

❏ Cholesterol free – Take care, the food may still be high in saturated fat.

❏ Fat reduced – But is it good fat? Compare saturated fat per 100 grams between products.

❏ No added sugar – Do you realise it could still raise your blood glucose?

❏ Lite – Light in what? It could mean simply light in colour.

Understanding nutrition information

To get the hard facts on the nutritional value of a food, look at the nutrition information table. Here you'll find the details regarding the fat, kilojoule, carbohydrate, fibre and sodium content of the food.

These are the key points to look for:

Energy – This is a measure of how many kilojoules or calories we get from a food. For a healthy diet we need to eat more foods with a low energy density in combination with smaller amounts of high energy dense foods.

To assess the energy density, look at the kilojoules per 100 grams. Solid foods with a low energy density contain less than 500 kilojoules per 100 grams.

Fat – Seek low saturated fat content, ideally less than 28 per cent of the total fat. For example, if the total fat content is 10 grams, you want saturated fat to be less than 2.8 grams. Strictly speaking, a food can be labelled as low in saturated fat if it contains less than 1.5 grams saturated fat per 100 grams.

Total carbohydrate – This is the starch plus any naturally occurring and added sugars in the food. There's no need to look at the sugar figure separately since it's the total carbohydrate that matters most.

You might check the total carb if you were monitoring your carbohydrate intake and to calculate the glycemic load of the serving. (See pages 49–50 for more information about the GL.)

Fibre – Most of us don't eat enough fibre so seek out foods that are high in fibre. A high-fibre food contains more than 1 gram of fibre per serving.

Sodium – This is a measure of the nasty part of salt in our food. Our bodies need some salt but most people consume far more than they need. Breads in particular tend to be high in sodium. Check the sodium content per 100 grams next time you buy – a low salt food contains less than 120 milligrams of sodium per 100 grams. Many packaged foods and convenience meals are well above this. Aim for less than 450 milligrams per 100 grams with these foods, or at least aim to consume higher sodium types infrequently.

Choose iodised salt, because Australians and New Zealanders are running low on iodine for optimum thyroid function.

 Look out for this shopping trolley icon for ways to cut your food budget and increase your healthy eating habits.

YOUR SHOPPING LIST

Build your own shopping list using our healthy suggestions as a framework. Look out for the GI symbol when shopping – your trusted guide to making healthy low GI choices.

The bakery

❏ Fruit loaf – dense with fruit and/or grains
❏ Low GI bread
    Wholegrain
    Wholegrain and seeds
    Wholemeal and oats
    Rye
    Genuine sourdough
    Soy and linseed
❏ Pita bread
❏ Low GI corn tortilla

The refrigerated cabinet

❏ Cheese
    Cottage cheese/ricotta, reduced fat
    Grated cheese, reduced fat
    Parmesan cheese
    Sliced cheese, reduced fat
❏ Dairy desserts
    Custard, low fat
    Fruche, low fat
❏ Dips
    Hommus

❏ Fruit juice

> Look for fruit juices that are '100% pure' and 'unsweetened'. And remember not to overdo it — one serve is 200 ml.

Apple juice

Cranberry juice

Grapefruit juice

Orange juice

❏ Margarine, canola or olive oil based

❏ Milk

Low fat

Low fat, flavoured

Skim

❏ Noodles, fresh

> Many Asian noodles, such as Hokkien, udon and rice vermicelli, have low to intermediate GI values because of their processing, whether they are made from wheat or rice flour.

❏ Pasta, fresh

Ravioli

Tortellini

❏ Soy products

Soy milk, low fat, calcium-enriched

Soy yoghurt

Soy frozen dessert

❏ Sushi

❏ Tofu

❏ Yoghurt

Low fat natural yoghurt provides the most calcium for the fewest kilojoules/calories. Have vanilla or fruit versions as a dessert, or use natural yoghurt as a condiment in savoury dishes.

Drinking yoghurt, low fat
Fruit or vanilla flavoured, low fat
Plain/natural, low fat

The freezer

❏ Frozen berries

Berries can make any dessert special. Using frozen ones means you don't have to wait until berry season.

Blueberries
Raspberries
Strawberries

❏ Frozen fruit desserts or gelato

❏ Frozen vegetables

Frozen vegetables are handy to add to a quick meal.

Beans
Broccoli
Cauliflower
Corn
Mixed vegetables
Peas

Spinach

Stir-fry mix

❑ Frozen yoghurt

Frozen yoghurt is a fantastic substitute for ice-cream. Some products even have a similar creamy texture, but with much less fat.

❑ Ice-cream

Vanilla or flavoured, reduced or low fat

Fresh fruit & vegetables

❑ Basics

Carrots

Chillies

Garlic

Ginger

Lemons or limes

Low GI potatoes, e.g. Carisma

Onions

Parsnips

Pumpkin

Sweet corn

Orange-fleshed sweet potato

Taro

Yam

❑ Fruit, fresh, depending on season

Apples

Apricots

    Grapefruit

    Grapes

    Mango

    Oranges

    Peaches

    Pears

    Strawberries

❏ Herbs, fresh, depending on season

> Fresh herbs are available in most supermarkets and there really is no substitute for the flavour they impart.

    Basil

    Chives

    Coriander

    Mint

    Parsley

❏ Leafy green and other seasonal vegetables

> Pile your plate high with leafy greens and eat your way to longterm health.

    Asian greens, such as bok choy

    Asparagus

    Beans

    Broccoli

    Brussels sprouts

    Cabbage

    Cauliflower

    Eggplant

    Fennel

Leeks

Mushrooms

Snowpeas

Spinach or silverbeet

Squash

Zucchini

❑ Salad vegetables, depending on season

Avocados

Bagged mixed salad greens

Capsicum

Celery

Cucumbers

Lettuce

Rocket

Spring onions

Sprouts, such as mung bean, snowpea, alfalfa

Tomatoes

General groceries

❑ Beverages

Coffee

Flavoured milk powders, such as Milo

Tea

❑ Breakfast cereals

Low GI packaged breakfast cereal

Natural muesli

Rolled oats, traditional

Besides their use in porridge, oats can be added
to cakes, biscuits, breads and desserts.

❑ Canned foods

    Baked beans

    Beans, such as cannellini, butter, borlotti, lima,
       kidney, chickpeas, Mexi-beans etc

    Corn kernels

    Four bean mix

    Lentils

    Tomatoes, whole, crushed

    Tomatoes can be used freely because they are
    rich in anti-oxidants, as well as having a low GI.

    Tomato paste

    Tomato soup

    Tuna, in spring water or oil

    Salmon, in water

    Sardines

    Skim milk, evaporated

    Canned, evaporated skim milk makes an
    excellent substitute for cream in pasta sauces.

❑ Canned fruit

    Have a variety of canned fruit on hand – choose brands
    labelled with 'no added sugar' fruit juice syrup.

    Mixed fruit salad

    Peaches

    Pears

❑ Cereals and wholegrains

Amaranth

A high protein ancient grain that can be used like rice.

Bulgur/cracked wheat
Use bulgur to make tabbouli, or add to vegetable burgers, stuffings, soups and stews.

Chia

Not strictly a grain, chia seeds (the richest plant source of omega-3) can be sprinkled on cereal, yoghurt or salads or ground and mixed with flour to lower the GI when making baked goods.

Couscous

Couscous can be ready in minutes; serve with casseroles and braised dishes. Israeli/toasted/pearl couscous are different from the instant variety and have a low GI.

Noodles
Oat biscuits
Pasta

Pasta is a great source of carbohydrates and B vitamins.

Pearl barley

One of the oldest cultivated cereals, barley is very nutritious and high in fibre. Look for products such as pearl barley to use in soups, stews and pilafs.

Rice, such as Basmati, SunRice Doongara low GI Clever rice or low GI brown rice

Quinoa

Quinoa cooks in about 10–15 minutes and has a slightly chewy texture. It can be used as a substitute for rice, couscous or bulgur wheat. It is very important to rinse the grains thoroughly before cooking.

❏ Condiments

Asian sauces

Hoisin, oyster, soy and fish sauces are a good range of Asian sauces.

Black pepper
Chilli, minced
Curry paste
Dried herbs
Garlic, minced
Ginger, minced
Horseradish cream
Mustard

Pasta sauce
Salt (iodised)
Soy sauce
Spices
Tomato sauce

❏ Dried fruit
Apple rings
Apricots
Prunes
Raisins
Sultanas

❏ Dried legumes
Beans

Keep a variety of beans in the cupboard including
cannellini, borlotti, lima, kidney, soy, pinto.

Chickpeas
Lentils
Split peas

❏ Deli items or pre-packed jars
Anchovies
Capers
Capsicum, chargrilled
Eggplant, chargrilled
Olives
Sundried tomatoes

❑ Eggs

Buy omega-3-enriched eggs. They are a good way of boosting your omega-3 intake, particularly if you don't eat fish.

❑ Nuts and seeds

Natural almonds, Brazil nuts, walnuts, cashews (unsalted), sesame seeds, pumpkin seeds, chia seeds, sunflower seeds

❑ Oils and vinegars

Canola or olive oil

Cooking spray, canola or olive oil

Use extra-virgin olive oil for salad dressings, marinades and dishes that benefit from its flavour.

Vinegar, balsamic and white wine

❑ Spreads

Honey

Avoid the honey blends, and use 'pure floral' honeys, which have a much lower GI.

Jam

A dollop of good-quality jam on toast contains fewer kilojoules than butter or margarine.

Peanut butter

Choose one made with 100% peanuts and no
other added oils.

Vegemite

Butcher/meat department

❏ Bacon

Bacon is a valuable ingredient in many dishes
because of the flavour it offers. You can make a
little bacon go a long way by trimming off all fat
and chopping it finely – look for bacon short cuts
where all the fat has been trimmed. Lean ham is
often a more economical and leaner way to go.

❏ Beef, lean
❏ Chicken
   Skinless chicken breast or drumsticks
❏ Fish
   Any type of fresh fish
❏ Ham, lean
❏ Lamb fillets, lean
❏ Minced beef, lean
❏ Pork fillets, lean

Shopping & storage tips

Cheese

Any reduced fat cheese is great to keep handy in the fridge. A block of parmesan is indispensable and will keep for up to a month. Reduced fat cottage and ricotta cheeses have a short life so are best bought as needed. They can be a good alternative to butter or margarine in a sandwich.

Vegetables & fruit

Vegetables are best fresh, so shop two or three times a week if you can and use them within a few days.

Ethylene gas produced by ageing fruit and vegetables leads to their deterioration. You can minimise the effect of ethylene by storing vegetables in the fridge in long-life bags, which are available in the food wrap section of supermarkets, or you can use special cartridges (available in some supermarkets) designed to absorb ethylene. Fruits give off more ethylene than vegetables, but vegetables are more sensitive to its effects, so if you have two crispers, keep fruit in one and vegetables in the other.

Legumes

Whether you buy them dried, or opt for canned convenience, you are choosing one of nature's lowest GI foods. They are high in fibre and packed with nutrients, providing protein, carbohydrate, B vitamins, folate and minerals. When you add legumes to meals and snacks, you reduce the overall GI of your diet because your body digests them slowly. This is primarily because their starch breaks down relatively slowly (or incompletely) during cooking and they contain tannins and enzyme inhibitors that also slow digestion.

Although they have an excellent shelf life, old beans take longer to cook than young, which is why it's a good idea to buy them from shops where you know turnover is brisk. Once home, store them in airtight containers in a cool, dry place – they will keep their colour better.

Preparing dried legumes

1. **Wash.** Wash thoroughly in a colander or sieve first, keeping an eye out for any small stones or 'foreign' material (especially with lentils).
2. **Soak.** Soaking plumps the beans, makes them softer and tastier, and reduces cooking time a little. Place them in a saucepan, cover with about three times their volume of cold water and soak overnight, or for at least four hours. As a rule of thumb, the larger the seed, the longer the soaking time required. There's no need to soak lentils or split peas.
3. **Cook.** Drain, rinse thoroughly, then add fresh water – two to three times the volume of the legumes. Bring to the boil then reduce the heat and simmer until tender. Generally, you will need to simmer lentils and peas for 45–60 minutes,

and beans and chickpeas for 1–2 hours, but check the recipe instructions. A couple of points to keep in mind:

❑ Adding salt to the water during cooking will slow down water absorption and the legumes will take longer to cook.

❑ Make sure that legumes are tender before you add acidic flavourings such as lemon juice or tomatoes. Once they are in an acid medium they won't get any softer no matter how long you cook them.

Time-saving tips:

❑ If you don't have time to soak legumes overnight, add three times the volume of water to rinsed beans, bring to the boil for a few minutes then remove from the heat and soak for an hour. Drain, rinse, add fresh water then cook as usual.

❑ Cooked legumes freeze well. Prepare a large quantity of beans or chickpeas and freeze in meal-sized batches to use as required.

❑ Store soaked or cooked beans in an airtight container in the fridge. They will keep for several days.

Noodles

You can buy noodles fresh, dried or boiled (wet). Fresh and boiled noodles will be in the refrigerated cabinets in your supermarket or Asian grocery store. Use them as soon as possible after purchase or store in the refrigerator for a day or two. Dried noodles are handy to have in the pantry for quick and easy meals in minutes. They will keep for several months, provided you haven't opened the packet. Egg noodles are made from wheat flour and eggs. They are readily available dried, and you can find fresh egg noodles in the refrigerator section of the supermarket or Asian grocery store. Hokkien noodles are 'wet' egg noodles and will be in the refrigerator section too. Instant noodles are usually precooked and dehydrated egg noodles. Check the label as they are sometimes fried.

Spices

Most spices, including ground cumin, turmeric, cinnamon, paprika and nutmeg, should be bought in small quantities because they lose pungency with age and incorrect storage. Keep them in dark, airtight containers.

Your shopping Q&A

How can I feed a big family with cost-effective, no-hassle low GI foods?

Feeding a big family on a budget can be hard. But low GI eating often means making a move back to the inexpensive, filling and healthy staple foods that our parents and grandparents enjoyed. This includes traditional oats for breakfast porridge, legumes such as beans, chickpeas and lentils (available in cans), cereal grains like barley, and of course plenty of fresh vegetables and fruit, which naturally have a low GI. Some of these foods may take a little more time to prepare than the high GI, processed, packaged, and pricey 'convenience' foods piled high on supermarket shelves, but the savings will be considerable and the health benefits immeasurable. For some easy food ideas to feed your family, check out *The Low GI Family Cookbook*.

I have recently been diagnosed with coeliac disease and/or gluten intolerance. Any suggestions for foods that are both low GI *and* wheat-free?

This is not as hard as you may think. If you like Asian food – Indian dhals, stir-fries with rice, sushi, noodles – you're in luck, because they are all low GI. Choose vermicelli noodles prepared from rice or mung beans, and low GI rices such as SunRice Low GI. Use sweet potato or Carisma potatoes instead of regular potato, use all manner of vegetables without any regard for their GI. Choose fruits for their low GI. If you can tolerate dairy products, then take advantage of them for their universal low GI. If lactose intolerance is a problem, reach for live cultured yoghurts and lactose-hydrolysed milks. Even ice-cream can be enjoyed if you ingest a few drops of lactase enzyme first.

I'm a very keen cook. If I make my own bread (or dumplings, pancakes, muffins etc), which flours, if any, are low GI?

There are no GI ratings for refined flour, whether it's made from wheat, soy or other grains. This is because the GI rating of a food must be tested physiologically, that is, in real people. So far we haven't had volunteers willing to tuck into 50 gram portions of raw flour! What we do know, however, is that bakery products such as scones, cakes, biscuits, doughnuts and pastries made from refined flour, whether it's white or wholemeal, are quickly digested and absorbed.

What should you do with your own baking? Try to increase the soluble fibre content by partially substituting flour with oat bran, rice bran or rolled oats, and increase the bulkiness of the product with dried fruit, nuts, muesli, All-Bran or unprocessed bran. Don't think of it as a challenge. It's an opportunity for some creative cooking. See some of our recipes in *The Low GI Family Cookbook*, *The Low GI Diet Cookbook* and *The Low GI Vegetarian Cookbook*.

Lower GI breads and breakfast cereals

Did you know that the type of bread and cereal you eat affects the overall GI of your diet the most? Why? Well, cereal grains such as rice, wheat, oats, barley and rye, and products made from them, such as bread and breakfast cereals, are the most concentrated sources of carbohydrate in our diet.

Here's a list of the lower GI breads and breakfast cereals you will find in your local supermarket.

Breads	GI
Bakers Delight	
Cape Seed Loaf	48
Wholemeal Country Grain	53
Bürgen	
Ⓖ Soy-Lin	52
Ⓖ Rye	53
Ⓖ Pumpkin Seeds	51
Ⓖ Wholemeal and Seeds	39
Ⓖ Fruit and Muesli	53
Ⓖ Wholegrains and Oat	51
Coles	
Ⓖ 7 Seeds & Grain Bread	45
Ⓖ In-store bakery, low GI sliced bread	51
Ⓖ High Fibre Low GI white sandwich loaf	55
Country Life	
Low GI Harvest Grain Gluten-Free White Bread	54
Golden Hearth	
Organic Heavy Wholegrain	53
Herman Brot	
Low carb bread	24
Mission Foods	
Ⓖ White corn tortillas	52
Pav's Allergy Bakery	
Spelt Multigrain	54

Breads	GI
Tip Top	
Ⓖ 9 Grain Original	53
Ⓖ 9 Grain Pumpkin Seed	52
Ⓖ 9 Grain Wholemeal	53
Spicy Fruit loaf	54

Breakfast cereals and bars	GI
Belvita Breakfast Biscuits	
Cranberry	40
Crunchy Oats	54
Fruit & Fibre	47
Honey & Nut with Choc Chips	46
Milk & Cereals	45
Be Natural	
Cashew, Almond, Hazelnut & Coconut Muesli	54
Multi-grain Porridge	51
Pink Lady Apple & Flame Raisin Muesli	51
Carman's Classic	
Cranberry & Apple Clusters	54
Deluxe Gluten-free Fruit Muesli	51
Fruit Muesli	42
Honey Roasted Nut Clusters	51
Natural Bircher Muesli	46
Original Recipe Fruit-Free Muesli	42
Coles	
Ⓖ Apricot, Almond & Date Muesli	44
Ⓖ Smart Buy Muesli	46
Ⓖ Summer Fruits Muesli	54
Ⓖ Vanilla Flavoured Oat Clusters	54
Freedom Foods	
Free Oats Crunchola	
Apple & Blueberry	54
Apple & Cinnamon	52
Berries & Vanilla	47
Gluten-Free Muesli	39
Hi-Lite Cereal	54
Yeast-Free Muesli	44

Breakfast cereals and bars	GI
Goodness Superfoods	
Digestive 1st	39
Fibreboost Sprinkles	34
Heart 1st	46
Protein 1st	36
Quick Sachets Barley & Oats 1st	
Apple & Honey Porridge	55
Traditional Barley & Oats 1st: Porridge	47
Kellogg's	
All-Bran, original	55
High Fibre Muesli: Almond & Apricot	
with Sultanas and Pepita	54
High Fibre Muesli: Cranberry & Pink Lady	
Apple with Pepita	49
Frosties	55
Guardian	34
Monster Muesli Company	
Multi-grain Porridge	55
Morning Sun	
⊙ Natural Style Muesli, Apricot and Almond	49
⊙ Natural Style Muesli, Peach and Pecan	49
⊙ Natural Style Muesli, Fruit Free Nuts and Seeds	55
Nestlé	
⊙ Milo Protein Clusters	47
Sanitarium	
Natural muesli	49
Uncle Tobys	
O&G Protein Crunchy Granola: Almond & Vanilla	48
O&G Protein Crunchy Granola: Cranberry,	
Hazelnut & Pepita	52
Vogel's	
Ultra Bran	45
Grain Clusters, Classic	54
Muesli, Cluster Spice	51
Muesli, Fruit & Nut	48

How do you know if it's truly low GI?

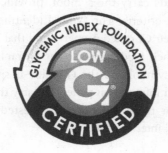

The GI symbol makes healthy shopping easier. This symbol means that the food has been assessed by the experts. And it's your guarantee that the GI value stated near the nutrition information table is accurate.

Foods that carry the certified GI symbol have also been judged against a range of nutrient criteria so you can be sure that the food is a healthy nutritional choice for its food group.

In the tables, you'll see that we have added a G beside the products that carry the GI symbol.

Why put the GI symbol on food labels?

Before 2001, people have had to rely on published lists of the glycemic index of foods to help them decide which carbohydrate foods to eat. The GI symbol helps identify healthy foods that have a GI value, making it much easier for you to choose foods on the basis of their GI.

Which foods carry the GI symbol?
Low GI foods carry the symbol, provided they meet the nutrient criteria. The symbol identifies foods that have had their GI tested properly, and that are a healthy choice for their food category. The GI ranking is stated within the symbol and the GI value is specified near the nutrition information panel. To carry the GI symbol the food has to be independently tested following a standardised international method.

Is the GI symbol an indication that foods are healthy?
Foods with the Glycemic Index symbol are healthy in other respects. To earn the certification, foods must be a good source of carbohydrate, and meet a host of other nutrient criteria including kilojoules, total and saturated fat, sodium (salt), and when appropriate, dietary fibre and calcium.

Are foods with the GI symbol good for people with diabetes?
In most cases the answer is yes. However, if you have diabetes you need to consider the quantity of carbohydrate in your serving of food, as well as the GI. Calculating the glycemic load (grams of carbohydrate × GI ÷100) is one way of combining both factors. (See pages 49–50 for more information on the GL.)

How can we be sure the information is accurate?

Foods in the program are required to undergo re-testing for their GI if there is any change in product formulation. All product labels and advertising that use the symbol or mention the program are pre-approved by the Glycemic Index Foundation. The Glycemic Index Foundation is not responsible, though, for the accuracy and legality of labels and marketing claims of the foods in the program.

Who is the Glycemic Index Foundation?

The Glycemic Index Foundation is a not-for-profit health promotion charity, supported by the University of Sydney and JDRF (Australia). It represents Australia's peak body of glycemic index research and education. Manufacturers pay the Glycemic Index Foundation a licence fee to use the certified GI symbol on their products and the income is channelled back into education and research.

Why don't all low GI foods have the symbol?

A food may make a low GI claim on its label, yet not carry the symbol. It may have been tested correctly (check the tables on pages 99–197 or the online database at www.glycemicindex.com, or contact the food manufacturer to double-check), but the manufacturer may choose not to participate in the GI Symbol Program. More likely, the food does not meet the other nutritional guidelines as it may be high in kilojoules, total or saturated fat, sodium, or low in fibre or calcium – check the nutrition information panel.

What about other labels that claim a food is low GI? Can I trust them?

Claims about the GI of foods were incorporated into the Australia New Zealand Food Standards Code in January 2013 and came into full effect in January 2015. Under this new legislation, in order to make a generic low GI claim, foods must have been tested according to Australian Standard 4694 – 2007 and also meet the requirements of Food Standards Australia New Zealand's Nutrient profiling scoring criterion. The GI value must also be included in the food's nutrition information panel so that the claim can be verified.

This new legislation should stop any false or misleading claims about GI being made on the labels of food sold in Australia and New Zealand as the legislation is enforceable. Contact your local Food Authority if you have any concerns.

You may also see products claiming to be 'low glycemic' or 'diabetic friendly' leaving it open as to whether it's low GI, low GL, or low carb. Be cautious with these claims as the product could actually be high in saturated fat (check the nutrition label). Manufacturers making these claims may not be intending to mislead the consumer, they simply may not understand the difference. It's useful to write and ask what they mean and where the food was tested. There are a number of foods that use low GI logos that are similar to the Certified Low Glycemic Index logo. Some of these cases have been pursued through legal channels.

❏ Consumers in Australia or New Zealand who have concerns about GI label claims should contact FSANZ and/or the Australian Competition and Consumer Commission (ACCC).

❏ Consumers in the US and Canada can contact the Food and Drug Administration's Office of Compliance at the Center for Food Safety and Applied Nutrition (for the US) and the Canadian Food Inspection Agency (for Canada).

For more information about the Glycemic Index Symbol Program and the latest list of approved products go to www.gisymbol.com

How we determine the GI value

The GI is a scale from 0 to 100 that captures how the carbohydrates in foods affect blood glucose levels ('glycemia'). It's based on testing real foods in real people. To make an absolutely fair comparison, all foods are tested following an internationally standardised method. The higher the GI, the higher the blood glucose levels after consumption of a standard amount. The GI rating of a food must be tested physiologically and only a few centres around the world currently provide a legitimate testing service.

Testing the GI of a food requires a group of ten volunteers and knowledge of the food's carbohydrate content. After an overnight fast, each subject consumes a portion of the test food containing a specified amount of carbohydrate (usually 50 grams, but sometimes 25 grams). Fingerprick blood samples are taken at 15- to 30-minute intervals over the next two hours. During this time, blood glucose levels rise and fall back to baseline levels. The full extent of glycemia (rise in blood glucose) is assessed by measuring the area under the curve using a computer algorithm.

There will be some variation between volunteers, but if we were to test them again and again, they all will tend to move towards the average of the whole group.

What is the GL?

Your blood glucose rises and falls when you eat a food or meal containing carbohydrate. How high it rises and how long it remains high depends on the quality of the carbohydrate (its glycemic index value or GI) as well as the quantity of carbohydrate in your meal. Researchers at Harvard University came up with a term that combines these two factors – glycemic load (GL).

Some people think that GL should be used instead of GI when comparing foods because it reflects the glycemic impact of both the quantity and quality of carbohydrate in a food. But more often than not, it's low GI (not low GL) that predicts good health outcomes, the reason being that following the low glycemic load (GL) route can lead you straight to a low carb diet: for example, fatty meats and butter have a low GL. But if you eat plenty of low GI foods, you'll find that you are automatically reducing the GL of your diet and, at the same time, you'll feel fuller for longer.

We also emphasise that there's no need to get overly technical about this. Think of the GI as a tool allowing you to choose one food over another in the same food group – the best bread to choose, the best cereal to choose etc – and don't get bogged down with figures. A low GI diet is about eating a wide variety of healthy foods that fuel our bodies best – on the whole these are the less processed and wholesome foods that will provide carbs in a slow release form.

Calculating the GL

The glycemic load is calculated simply by multiplying the GI value of a food by the amount of carbohydrate per serving and dividing by 100.

Here's how:

$$\text{Glycemic load} = (\text{GI} \times \text{carbohydrate per serving}) \div 100$$

Let's say you wanted to have an apple for a snack. Apples have a GI of 38 and 1 medium apple contains 15 grams of carbohydrate. So, the glycemic load of your apple snack is $(38 \times 15) \div 100 = 6$.

If you were very hungry and tucked into 2 apples you would be eating 30 grams of carbs and the GL of your snack would be 12. The GI doesn't change, but you are eating more carbs because you are eating 2 apples.

Low GI
eating out

Eating out the low GI way

Whether you think it is compatible with healthy eating or not, statistics tell us that at some point you are going to be eating out or buying takeaway food. Eating out can really test your resolve as far as healthy eating goes. Like any food choice, however, the more often we eat out, the more important it is that we choose healthy options. If you only eat out once a month you needn't be too fussy, but if it's three to four times a week, good choices are critical.

Finding the low GI choice on the menu
Indian food

The traditional accompaniment for Indian dishes is steamed Basmati rice, which is a classic low GI choice. Lentil dhal offers another lower GI accompaniment, but make sure they don't add the oil topping (tadka).

Unleavened breads such as chapatti or roti may have a lower GI than normal bread but they will boost the carbohydrate content of the meal and increase the GL.

Our suggestions:

❑ Tikka (dry roasted) or tandoori (marinated in spices and yoghurt) chicken

❑ Basmati rice

❑ Cucumber raita

❑ Spicy spinach (saag).

Japanese food

Sushi has a low GI, and any refrigerated rice has a lower GI than when it is freshly cooked. The vinegar used in preparation of sushi helps keep the GI low (acidity helps slow stomach emptying), and so do the viscous fibres in the seaweed. Typical ingredients and flavours to enjoy are shoyu (Japanese soy sauce), mirin (rice wine), wasabi (a strong horseradish), miso (soybean paste), pickled ginger (oshinko), sesame seeds and sesame oil. Go easy on deep-fried dishes such as tempura.

Japanese restaurants are great places to stock up on omega-3 fats, as dishes such as sushi and sashimi made with salmon and tuna contain high amounts of beneficial polyunsaturated fatty acids.

Our suggestions:

❏ Miso soup

❏ Edamame

❏ Sushi

❏ Teppanyaki (steak, seafood and vegetables)

❏ Yakitori (skewered chicken and onions in teriyaki sauce)

❏ Sashimi (thinly sliced raw fish or beef)

❏ Shabu-shabu (thin slices of beef quickly cooked with mushrooms, cabbage and other vegetables)

❏ Side orders such as seaweed salad, wasabi, soy sauce and pickled ginger.

Thai food

Thai food is generally sweet and spicy and contains aromatic ingredients such as basil, lemongrass and galangal. Spicy Thai salads which usually contain seafood, chicken or meat are a delicious light meal. For starters, avoid the deep-fried items such as spring rolls.

One downside to Thai cuisine is the coconut milk, which really raises the saturated fat content of Thai curry. So don't feel you have to consume all of the sauce or soup. The traditional accompaniment to Thai food is plain, steamed jasmine rice, but this is very high GI so you are better off if you can reduce the quantity. Noodles are always on the menu as well, but avoid fried versions. Boiled rice noodles may be an option. Limit yourself to a small helping or, if you are having takeaway, you could cook up some Doongara rice at home as an accompaniment.

Our suggestions:

❑ Tom yum – hot and sour soup

❑ Thai beef or chicken salad

❑ Wok-tossed meats or seafood

❑ Stir-fried mixed vegetables

❑ Small serve of steamed noodles or rice

❑ Fresh spring rolls (not fried).

Italian food

The big plus with Italian restaurants is the supply of low GI pasta with an array of sauces. Good choices are arrabiata, puttanesca, Napoletana and marinara sauces (without cream). Despite what you may think, most Italians don't sit down to huge bowls of pasta, so don't be afraid to leave some on your plate (or order an entrée size) – the GI may be low but a large serve of pasta will have a high GL. Other good choices include minestrone and vegetable dishes, lean veal and grilled seafood. Steer clear of crumbed and deep-fried seafood.

Our suggestions:

❑ Minestrone

❑ Veal escalopes in tomato-based sauce

❑ Prosciutto (paper-thin slices of smoky ham) wrapped around melon

❑ Barbecued or grilled seafood such as calamari or octopus

❑ Roasted or chargrilled fillet of beef, lamb loin or poultry

❑ Green garden salad with olive oil and balsamic vinegar

❑ Sorbet, gelato or simply a fresh fruit platter

❑ Entrée-size pasta with seafood and tomato or stock-based sauce.

Greek and Middle Eastern food

In Mediterranean cuisine, olive oil, lemon, garlic and onions and other vegetables abound. Many dishes are chargrilled and specialities such as barbecued octopus or grilled sardines are excellent choices. You will find regular bread replaced with flat bread or Turkish bread, while potatoes are replaced with wholegrains such as bulgur (in tabbouli) and couscous. Among the small appetising mezze dishes, you could pick and choose what you like. Many of the choices are healthy, such as hommus, baba ghanoush, olives, tzatziki and dolmades.

Our suggestions:

❏ Mezze platter with Lebanese bread

❏ Souvlaki (chargrilled skewers of meat with vegetables)

❏ Kofta (balls of minced lamb with bulgur wheat)

❏ Greek salad of fresh lettuce, tomato, olives, feta and capsicum, with balsamic dressing or oil and lemon

❏ Fresh fruit platter

❏ Falafel with tabbouli and hommus with a flat bread.

Tips for those who routinely eat at restaurants

1. *Walk* to the restaurant if possible.
2. Order water as soon as you arrive.
3. Send the bread basket away (unless it's *exceptional*).
4. Order green salad, oysters au naturel or soup for entrée.
5. Order an entrée for your main course (or specify entrée size).
6. Alternatively, eat *only half* of everything on your plate.
7. Tell the waiter to hold the hot chips.
8. Share dessert with a dining companion.
9. Drink no more than one or two glasses of alcohol.
10. Walk back to the office or climb the stairs.

Fast-food outlets
Burgers and French fries are a bad idea – quickly eaten, high in saturated fat and rapidly absorbed high GI carbs that fill you with kilojoules that don't last long. Some fast-food chains are introducing healthier choices but read the fine print. Look out for lean protein, low GI carbs, good fats and lots of vegetables.

Our suggestions:

❑ Marinated and barbecued chicken, rather than fried

❑ Salads such as coleslaw or garden salad; eat the salad first

❑ Corn on the cob as a healthy side order

❑ Individual menu items rather than meal deals – never upsize.

Lunch bars
Steer clear of places displaying lots of deep-fried fare and head towards fresh food bars offering fruit and vegetables. Tubs of garden or Greek salad finished with fruit and yoghurt make a healthy, low GI choice.

With sandwiches and melts, choose the fillings carefully. Including cheese can make the fat exceed 20 grams per sandwich (that's as much as chips!). Make sure you include some vegetables or salad in, or alongside, the sandwich.

Our suggestions:

❏ Dense grain bread rather than white

❏ Salad fillings for sandwiches, or as a side order instead of fries

❏ Pasta dishes with both vegetables and meat

❏ Lebanese kebabs with tabbouli and hommus

❏ Grilled fish rather than fried

❏ Vegetarian pizza

❏ Gourmet wraps.

Cafés

Whether it's a quick snack or a main meal, catching up with a friend for coffee doesn't have to tip your diet off balance. Pass on breads, but if you really must, something like a dense Italian bread is better than a garlic or herb bread.

Whatever you order, specify: 'no French fries – extra salad instead' so temptation does not confront you. If you want something sweet, try a skim iced chocolate or a single little biscuit or slice.

Our suggestions:

❏ Skim milk coffee rather than full cream milk

❏ Sourdough or wholegrain bread instead of white or wholemeal

❏ Bruschetta with tomatoes, onions, olive oil and basil on a dense Italian bread rather than buttery herb or garlic bread

❏ Salad as a main or side order, with the dressing served separately so you control the amount

❏ Chargrilled steak or chicken breast rather than fried or crumbed

❏ Vegetable-topped pizza – such as capsicum, onion, mushroom, artichoke, eggplant

❏ Lean meat pizza – such as ham, fresh seafood or sliced chicken breast

❏ Pasta with sauces such as marinara, Bolognese, Napoletana, arrabiata (tomato with olives, roasted capsicum and chilli), and piccolo (eggplant, roasted capsicum and artichoke)

❏ Seafood such as marinated calamari, grilled with chilli and lemon or steamed mussels with a tomato sauce

❏ Water, mineral water or freshly squeezed fruit and vegetable juices rather than soft drinks.

Asian meals

Asian meals including Chinese, Thai, Indian and Japanese offer a great variety of foods, making it possible to select a healthy meal with some careful choices.

Keeping in line with the 1, 2, 3 steps to a balanced meal (see page 8), seek out a lower GI carb such as Basmati rice, dhal, sushi or noodles. Chinese and Thai rice will traditionally be jasmine and although high GI, a small serve of steamed rice is better for you than fried rice or noodles.

Next add some protein – marinated tofu (bean curd), stir-fried seafood, Tandoori chicken, fish tikka or a braised dish with vegetables. Be cautious with pork and duck, for which fattier cuts are often used; and avoid Thai curries and dishes made with coconut milk because it's high in saturated fat.

And don't forget, the third dish to order is stir-fried vegetables!

Our suggestions:

❑ Steamed dumplings, dim sims or fresh spring rolls rather than fried entrées

❑ Clear soups to fill you up, rather than high-fat laksa

❑ Noodles in soups rather than fried in dishes such as pad Thai

❑ Noodle and vegetable stir-fries – if you ask for extra vegetables you may find that the one dish feeds two

❑ Seafood braised in a sauce with vegetables

❑ Tofu, chicken, beef, lamb or pork fillet braised with nuts, vegetables, black bean or other sauces

❑ Salads such as Thai salads

❑ Smaller serves of rice

❑ Vegetable dishes such as stir-fried vegetables, vegetable curry, dhal, channa (a delicious chickpea curry), and side orders such as pickles, cucumber and yoghurt, tomato and onion.

Airlines and airports

Airports are notoriously bad places to eat. Fast-food chains, a limited range, pre-made sandwiches, sad-looking cakes, a lack of fresh fruit and vegetables – and it's all expensive!

In airline lounges you will do better, although again, the range is limited. Fresh fruit is always on offer and usually some sort of vegetables, either as salad or soup. The bread is usually the super-high GI white French type and with crackers as the only other option, so you would do better to rely on fruit, fruit juices, yoghurt or a skim milk coffee for your carbs.

In-flight, unless you have the privilege of a sky chef, meals are fairly standard fare, including a salad and fruit if you're lucky. Many airlines offer special diets with advance bookings and although there's no guarantee it will meet your nutritional criteria, it may be healthier than what everyone else is having.

Travelling domestic economy these days, it's probably best to eat before you leave, take your own snacks with you, and decline the in-flight snack. (You really will be better off without that mini chocolate bar, biscuit, cake or muffin, which on some airlines you have to pay for.)

Our suggestions:

❏ Fresh fruit, soup and salad items in airline lounges rather than white bread, cheese, cakes and salami

- Small meals in-flight, rather than eating everything put in front of you
- Water to drink, wherever you are
- Dried fruit, nut bars, bananas or apples that you have taken along yourself.

Gluten-free eating out

Eating out on a gluten-free diet can be difficult, particularly as there is often gluten in items such as sauces, stock, dressings and gravy. It is important that the restaurant understands your need for a meal that is completely free of gluten and it may be a good idea to call beforehand to ensure that they can accommodate your needs.

Your state coeliac society should be able to give you a list of recommended restaurants to eat at, where you can be confident that they are able to provide you with a gluten-free meal. These are good places to start. Otherwise you need to ask plenty of questions and remember that, if you are in doubt, you are best to leave it out!

Following are some tips to making low GI gluten-free meal choices when eating out.

- Plain grilled steak, chicken or fish with a cob of sweet corn, and salad or steamed vegetables
- Indian dhal with Basmati rice
- Mexican tacos (if 100 per cent corn) with beans, salad, avocado, salsa and grated cheese
- Sushi filled with raw fish or avocado and cucumber (add pickled ginger and skip the soy sauce)

❏ Vietnamese rice paper rolls (but hold the dipping
sauce unless you can check if it is gluten-free)

❏ Asian rice noodles stir-fried with vegetables, tofu or
prawns, peanuts, coriander and lemon or lime juice
(check the sauces)

❏ Mixed-bean, chickpea or lentil salads (leave the
dressing unless you can check it is gluten-free)

❏ Falafel (check they are gluten-free) with hommus
and salad.

Low GI
gluten-free eating

Gluten-free eating

There is much more to a gluten-free lifestyle than focusing on foods you need to avoid. Eating well is the key to good health for everyone and eating the right foods gives your body the fuel it needs to perform at its best and the energy to get through the day. It's also an important part of managing and preventing other longterm health problems, including diabetes, heart disease, cancer and a range of digestive problems.

If you have coeliac disease and need to follow a strict gluten-free diet, we suggest that you join your state coeliac society and take advantage of the up-to-date and comprehensive information they provide for their members on shopping, cooking and eating gluten-free. Recent research has also found that some people are sensitive to gluten yet not allergic (as in coeliac disease). Symptoms include bloating, flatulence and lethargy. Gluten-free diets have been found to be helpful.

While it is great to see an increasing range of gluten-free foods making life easier for those with coeliac disease, unfortunately many of them are highly processed and some are high in fat and added sugar – two ingredients that are naturally gluten-free!

What is gluten?

Gluten is the protein found in the grains, wheat, rye, barley and triticale. Oats are frequently grown, harvested, milled and processed alongside gluten-containing grains, so they may be contaminated with gluten. They also contain a gluten-like protein which some people with coeliac disease react to. So, while research is ongoing, oats are currently not recommended for people with coeliac disease.

Gluten-free diets also tend to have a high glycemic index (GI). This is because many low GI staples such as whole wheat kernel breads, pasta, barley and oats are eliminated because they contain gluten. The gluten-free alternatives, due to their ingredients and processing methods, are often quickly digested and absorbed, raising blood glucose and insulin levels, and leaving you feeling hungry and often low on energy a few hours after eating. What this means in practice is that many people following a gluten-free diet are rarely satisfied after meals and may feel hungry between meals, which can lead to overeating and weight gain.

In addition, adults and children on a gluten-free diet can miss out on the numerous health benefits of:

❏ Getting enough fibre

❏ Managing blood glucose levels with low GI foods.
  (See the benefits of a low GI diet on page 3.)

Even on a wheat-free or gluten-free diet, you'll find that there are many low GI gluten-free foods you can enjoy in four of the five food groups:

❑ Virtually all fruits and vegetables

❑ Whole kernel grains in the breads and cereals group

❑ Legumes of all types in the meat and alternatives group

❑ Milk and yoghurt among the dairy foods.

There are a number of gluten-free breads, breakfast cereals, snack foods and pastas on the market. As not many have been GI tested, here are some guidelines for selecting lower GI options.

Bread
At the time of publication, we found only a limited range of low GI breads on the supermarket shelves.

Most of the gluten-free breads tested, including rolls and wraps, have been found to have a high GI. But here is a tip: check out the ingredients list and opt for breads that include chickpea- or legume-based flours and psyllium. For example, we know that chapattis made with besan (chickpea flour) have a low GI. If you make your own bread, try adding buckwheat kernels, rice bran and psyllium husks to lower the GI.

Breakfast cereals

Freedom Foods muesli and Vogel's fruit and nut muesli cereal both have a low GI. Rice bran and buckwheat kernels also have a low GI and can be used with other ingredients to make your own gluten-free muesli.

Most gluten-free breakfast cereals, including rice, buckwheat or millet puffs and flakes, have a moderate or high GI because they are refined, not wholegrain, foods. But you can reduce the GI if you serve them with fruit and yoghurt and a teaspoon or two of psyllium to boost the fibre. If you like cooked cereal, try quinoa porridge (made from whole quinoa grains) or make your own rice porridge (from a lower GI rice). Add psyllium husks and rice bran, along with fruit and low fat milk or yoghurt.

Noodles and pasta

There are several low GI, gluten-free options available in both fresh and dried varieties:

❑ Soba noodles, made from buckwheat

❑ Cellophane noodles, also known as Lungkow bean thread noodles or green bean vermicelli, made from mung bean flour

❑ Rice noodles, made from ground or pounded rice flour.

Most gluten-free pastas based on rice and corn (maize) tend to have moderate to high GI values (Coles' low GI pasta varieties being an exception). So opt for pastas made from legumes or soy – although they may be harder to find.

Whole cereal grains

Low GI cereal grains for those on a gluten-free diet include buckwheat, quinoa, and some varieties of rice and sweet corn. Currently there are no published values for amaranth, sorghum and teff. Millet has a high GI.

Rice

Rice can have a very high GI value, or a moderate one, depending on the variety and its amylose content. Instant and quick-cooking rices all tend to have a high GI. So, if you are a big rice eater, opt for the lower GI varieties with a higher amylose content such as Basmati rice (GI 58) or SunRice Doongara low GI Clever white or brown rice (GI 54).

Brown rice is an extremely nutritious form of rice and contains several B-group vitamins, minerals, dietary fibre and protein. The varieties tested to date tend to have a moderate or high GI (SunRice low GI varieties excepted), so try to combine this nourishing food with low GI ingredients like lentils or beans, or even in combination with wild rice.

Wild rice (GI 57) is not rice at all, but a type of grass seed. Arborio rice, used mainly in risotto, releases its starch during cooking and has a medium GI.

Legumes (pulses)

Dried or canned legumes, including beans, chickpeas and lentils, are among nature's lowest GI foods. They are high in fibre and packed with nutrients, providing

protein, carbohydrate, B vitamins, folate and minerals.
Check canned varieties for gluten content.

Nuts
Although nuts are high in fat (averaging around 50 per
cent of their content), it is largely unsaturated, so they
make a healthy substitute for snacks such as biscuits,
cakes, pastries, potato chips and chocolate. They also
contain relatively little carbohydrate, so most do not have
a GI value. Peanuts and cashews have very low GI values.
Avoid the varieties that are salted and cooked in oil –
choose raw and unsalted. Also be aware that dry-roasted
nuts may contain gluten.

Chestnuts are quite different from other nuts in that
they are low in fat and higher in carbohydrate. Naturally
gluten-free, they have recently been found to have a
low GI, which makes them a great low GI, high-fibre
carbohydrate food.

Low fat dairy foods and calcium-enriched soy products
Low fat varieties of milk, yoghurt and ice-cream, or
calcium-enriched soy alternatives, provide you with
sustained energy, boosting your calcium intake but not
your saturated fat intake. Check the labels of yoghurts,
ice-creams and soy milks, as some contain wheat-based
maltodextrins, which should be avoided.

Cheese is a good source of calcium, but it is a protein
food, not a carbohydrate – its lactose is drawn off in
the whey during production. This means that GI is not

relevant to cheese. Although perfect for sandwich fillings, snacks, and toppings for gratin dishes, remember that cheese can also contribute a fair number of kilojoules. Most cheese is around 30 per cent fat, much of it saturated. Ricotta and cottage cheese are good low fat choices.

For more information about coeliac disease and gluten intolerance plus more than 80 recipes, check out *The Low GI Guide to Gluten-free Cooking*.

Our favourite gluten-free food websites

www.coeliacsociety.com.au

www.glutenfreeshop.com.au

www.coeliac.org.nz

www.glutenfreegoodies.co.nz

Sugars & sweeteners

Sugars & sweeteners

Do you feel guilty every time you enjoy something sweet? Do you think diabetes equals no sugar? Join the club. Many people think that if something tastes good, it must be bad for them. And many people with diabetes, and even their doctors, mistakenly believe that sugar consumption is the most important explanation for high blood glucose readings.

While we now know that's not the case, old habits die hard. Traditionally, people with diabetes have been told to replace all sugar with an artificial sweetener and to drink diet soft drinks. It's enough to make some people with diabetes turn their backs on all dietary advice.

But wanting something sweet is instinctive, and hard to ignore. It is part of our 'hardwiring'. In our hunter-gatherer past, fruits, berries and honey were our only source of carbohydrate. Starch was harder to come by.

You'll be relieved to know that most diabetes organisations all around the world no longer advise strict avoidance of refined sugar or sugary foods. This is one of the happy spin-offs from research on the GI – recognition that both sugary foods and starchy foods raise your blood glucose.

Furthermore, scores of studies indicate that moderate amounts of added sugar in diabetic diets (for example 30–50 grams per day) does not result in either poor control or weight gain. Yes, a soft drink can be a concentrated source of kilojoules, but so can a fruit juice or an alcoholic drink.

You can enjoy refined or 'added' sugar in moderation – for example, a smear of jam on toast, a teaspoon of sugar in tea or coffee, a squeeze of honey on porridge, or a sweetened yoghurt. Even the World Health Organization says 'a moderate intake of sugar-rich foods can provide for a palatable and nutritious diet'. So forget the guilt trip and allow yourself the pleasure of sweetness.

Should we be concerned about fructose?

One form of sugar, fructose or fruit sugar, has been hitting the headlines because of the alarmist view that it is 'toxic' to our metabolism and should be consumed in minimal amounts. We don't agree and neither do the experts! Indeed, we believe that avoiding fructose could do more harm than good.

Fructose represents about half the natural sugars in fruit, vegetables and grains. It is also one half of the sucrose molecule (that's the one in cane or refined sugar) and as much as 70 per cent of the total sugars in honey. Fructose has a low GI (about 20) and in normal quantities it contributes to better diabetes control and lower blood pressure.

In Australia and New Zealand, average fructose consumption from all sources is less than 55 grams a day (14 teaspoons) with even the highest consumers eating less than 70 grams (17 teaspoons). Nutritional analysis of a typical low GI menu generates 70 grams of sugar (naturally occurring plus added) per day, of which 25–30 grams would be fructose.

Can fructose contribute to weight gain?

Of course! Like all carbohydrates, it contains 4 calories per gram, yet that's a lot less than the calories in a gram of fat (9 calories per gram) or alcohol (7 calories per gram). Recent expert reviews of all available human research on fructose concluded that fructose does not cause weight gain when it is substituted for other carbohydrates in diets providing similar calories. Consuming fructose *at very high doses* (more than 100 grams or 25 teaspoons per day) that provides excess calories may modestly increase body weight, but this effect is most likely due to the extra calories rather than the fructose.

From an evolutionary perspective, fructose was an important component of intelligent primate diets. Our human ancestors adored sweet berries and honey and made sweet drinks using both honey and floral nectars. In the 1980s, we analysed hundreds of traditional Aboriginal bushfoods, including sugarbag (bush honey) and dried bush fruits, such as the bush tomato *Solanum central*, which is 80 per cent (by weight) sugar. In other parts of the world, apiculture, the art of raising bees, was widely practised, even by the poor. Indeed at certain times in history, consumption of honey may well have rivalled our current consumption of refined sugar.

Strict avoidance of sugars and fructose reduces the enjoyment and quality of life for millions of people who enjoy a 'spoonful of sugar'. The take-home message is that a moderate consumption of fructose is compatible with a palatable and nutritious diet.

What about alternative sweeteners?

Alternatives to sugar are widely used by people with diabetes to sweeten drinks (tea and coffee) and foods (breakfast cereals); to sweeten recipes (for cakes and desserts); and in low kilojoule commercial products (soft drinks, cordials, jams, jellies and yoghurts).

They give sweetness with fewer kilojoules, and usually with less effect on blood glucose levels.

Not all alternative sweeteners are the same – some have just as many kilojoules as sugar, others have no kilojoules at all; some are thousands (yes thousands) of times sweeter than sugar; others are not very sweet at all. One thing they all have in common, however, is that they are more expensive than sugar.

There are lots of brands of sweeteners on the supermarket shelves, but essentially there are two main types:

❏ Nutritive sweeteners, and

❏ Non-nutritive sweeteners.

What's the difference?

Nutritive sweeteners

Nutritive sweeteners are simply those that provide some kilojoules and, as the name suggests, nutrients. Sugar, for example, is a nutritive sweetener, but so are things like sorbitol and maltodextrin. They have differing effects on blood glucose levels.

Old-fashioned table sugar stands up well under scrutiny – it is the second sweetest after fructose, has only a moderate GI, is the best value for money and is the easiest to use in cooking. And because it generally has a lower GI than the refined flour used in baking, it can actually lower the GI of many recipes! Less refined sweeteners like raw sugar, LoGiCane, honey, golden syrup and pure (100 per cent) maple syrup also provide very small amounts of calcium, potassium and magnesium.

The sugar alcohols, such as sorbitol, mannitol and maltitol, are generally not as sweet as table sugar, provide fewer kilojoules and have less of an impact on blood glucose levels. To overcome their lack of sweetness, food manufacturers usually combine them with non-nutritive sweeteners to help keep the kilojoule count down and minimise the effect on blood glucose levels. They will appear in the ingredients list on the food label.

The nutritive sweeteners such as sorbitol, mannitol, xylitol, erythritol and maltitol, and maltitol syrup, may have a laxative effect or cause wind or diarrhoea if you consume them in large amounts. Foods that contain more than 10 grams per 100 grams of these alternative sweeteners, or more than 25 grams per 100 grams of sorbitol, isomalt, or polydextrose, carry warning statements about the possible laxative effect on their labels. These products can be a particular problem for children and adolescents, because of their smaller body size.

Used in sensible quantities, fructose certainly rivals table sugar as a good all-round sweetener. It stands out from the crowd, being nearly twice as sweet as sugar, providing the same number of kilojoules, but having only one-third the GI, so you can use less fructose to achieve the same level of sweetness and as a result consume fewer kilojoules and experience a much smaller rise in your blood glucose levels. Its main drawback is cost.

If you have read alarmist reports about fructose and blood fats and/or insulin resistance, remember that most of this research was on rats and mice fed excessive quantities of pure added fructose – more than someone with even the sweetest tooth could tolerate. There is no evidence that fructose has adverse effects in people with diabetes consuming normal quantities e.g. less than 100 grams of added fructose per day. Average added fructose consumption is less than 30 grams per day in Australia. Most of it comes from added sucrose, which is half fructose and half glucose.

Non-nutritive sweeteners

Non-nutritive sweeteners (such as Equal, Splenda or saccharin) are all much sweeter than table sugar and essentially have no effect on your blood glucose levels because most are used in such small quantities and are either not absorbed into or metabolised by the body. Because they are only used in minute amounts, the number of kilojoules they provide is insignificant.

What's best to use for cooking?

The non-nutritive sweeteners that are made of protein molecules often break down when heated at high temperatures for long periods, thus losing their sweetness.

For this reason, they are not always ideal for baking. The best non-nutritive sweeteners to cook with are Splenda, and saccharin, and to a lesser extent Equal Spoonful.

Are they safe?

As a group, non-nutritive sweeteners have been studied more thoroughly than any other type of food additive. Questions about the safety of saccharin were raised when it was first discovered over 125 years ago, and its effect on human health has been monitored ever since. The same is true of more recent sweeteners such as aspartame and sucralose. There is no convincing evidence so far that any of the non-nutritive sweeteners on the market have any negative effects on our health.

While the non-nutritive sweeteners available in Australia and New Zealand are considered safe for everyone, some health professionals opt for caution and recommend that pregnant women avoid saccharin and cyclamate. This is because both of them cross the placenta to the growing fetus and can also be found in breast milk.

Also, studies in rats have shown an increased risk of bladder cancer due to saccharin use and kidney disease due to cyclamate use. To put this in perspective, remember that saccharin and cyclamate were both used widely after World War II because there was a worldwide sugar shortage, and we did not see an increase in bladder or kidney cancer over that period. So it seems unlikely that either sweetener is a problem for pregnant women or those who are breastfeeding. However, some women still choose to avoid these two non-nutritive sweeteners.

Stevia and monk fruit

Stevia has become popular with people seeking a more 'natural' alternative sweetener. Its natural reputation stems from the fact that it is derived from a sweet-tasting herb (*Stevia rebaudiana*) although stevia sweetener comes from a highly purified part of the plant (steviol glycosides). The leaves of the herb can be used as a sweetener themselves and in the dried form less than 2 tablespoons of crushed leaves can replace the sweetness of about 1 cup of sugar. In commercial powdered products the steviol glycosides are usually combined with other substances to provide bulk or improve taste and texture.

Monk fruit (also known as *luo han guo*), from Central Asia, is more recently being used as another source of a 'natural' alternative sweetener. It is available in Australia in a granular form under the brand name Norbu. Norbu is a sweet extract of the monk fruit in combination with a sugar alcohol as a carrier or bulking agent.

You can buy stevia in purified liquid and powder form and also in combination with other sugar substitutes in tablet, powdered, and granulated form. It is suitable for cooking. Commercially you will find it in a growing number of dairy foods, baked goods, confectionery and drinks, appearing as number 960 in the ingredient list.

Both are virtually calorie free, tooth-friendly and have no impact on blood glucose levels.

Phenylketonuria and aspartame

Foods and beverages in Australia and New Zealand that contain aspartame must carry a warning for people with phenylketonuria. Phenylketonuria is a rare genetic disease, which is characterised by an inability of the body to utilise the essential amino acid, phenylalanine. In Australia for example, about 1 in 10,000 newborn babies is affected with the condition. Managing this disease includes sticking to a low protein diet with particular emphasis on avoiding foods high in phenylalanine. As aspartame contains a significant amount of phenylalanine, it is not recommended for people with phenylketonuria.

The take-home message

Alternative sweeteners have been around for a very long time but have had little impact on the rate of obesity. In fact there is insufficient evidence to suggest that they benefit body weight, energy balance, appetite control, intake of carbohydrates, or cardiovascular risk factors.

If there are places in your diet where you are consuming large amounts of added sugar, you may benefit from replacing this with an alternative non-nutritive sweetener. For the rest of the time, just have a teaspoon or two of sugar and enjoy it.

Authorities such as Diabetes Australia and Diabetes New Zealand always recommend that people use a variety of sweeteners, including aspartame (951), sucralose (955), acesulphame K (950), and saccharin (954), so that the likelihood of excessive consumption of any one sweetener is reduced.

Nutritive sweeteners

Fructose
GI 19
16 kJ (4 Calories) per gram
46 kJ (11 Calories) per
teaspoon table sugar
equivalent*
Brand names: Fruisana

Fructose or fruit sugar has a relatively small effect on blood glucose levels. It is nearly twice as sweet as table sugar, but has the same amount of kilojoules per gram.
Sweetness relative to table sugar = 1.73 times more

Glucose
GI 100
16 kJ (4 Calories) per gram
108 kJ (26 Calories) per
teaspoon table sugar
equivalent*
Brand names: Glucodin;
Lucozade

Glucose is the sugar found in blood. When eaten, it causes blood glucose levels to rise rapidly. It is not as sweet as table sugar, but has the same amount of kilojoules.
Sweetness relative to table sugar = 0.74 times less

Golden syrup
GI 63
12 kJ (3 Calories) per gram
45 kJ (11 Calories) per
teaspoon table sugar
equivalent*

Golden syrup has a moderate effect on blood glucose levels, very similar to table sugar. It is sweeter than table sugar, and has less kilojoules.
Sweetness relative to table sugar = 1.33 times more

Honey
GI range 35–64
16 kJ (4 Calories) per gram
83 kJ (20 Calories) per
teaspoon table sugar
equivalent*

Honey has a moderate effect on blood glucose levels depending on whether it is a blend or a pure floral honey. The pure floral honeys appear to have lower GIs. On average, honey is slightly less sweet than table sugar, but has the same amount of kilojoules. Sweetness relative to table sugar = 0.97 times less

Isomalt
GI 60
11 kJ per gram
110 kJ per teaspoon table
sugar equivalent*
Food additive code number
953 (Australia/New Zealand)

Isomalt is very poorly absorbed, so it has essentially no effect on blood glucose levels when consumed in typical amounts. It is only half as sweet as table sugar, but has less kilojoules, and may have a laxative effect if eaten in large quantities. Sweetness relative to table sugar = 0.50 times less

Lactose
GI 46
16 kJ (4 Calories) per gram
500 kJ (120 Calories)
per teaspoon table sugar
equivalent*

Lactose is the sugar found in milk. When eaten, it causes blood glucose levels to rise slowly. It is not very sweet at all, but has the same amount of kilojoules as table sugar. Sweetness relative to table sugar = 0.16 times less

Maltitol
GI 69
13kJ (3 Calories) per gram
87 kJ (21 Calories) per
teaspoon table sugar
equivalent*
Food additive code 967
(Australia/New Zealand)

Maltitol is poorly absorbed,
so it has little effect on
blood glucose levels when
consumed in typical amounts.
It is only three-quarters as
sweet as table sugar, and
has the same amount of
kilojoules, and may have a
laxative effect if eaten in large
quantities.
Sweetness relative to table
sugar = 0.75 times less

Maltodextrins
GI not known
16 kJ (4 Calories) per gram
146 kJ (35 Calories) per
teaspoon table sugar
equivalent*

Maltodextrins are short chain
glucose polymers with a GI
similar to that of glucose. They
are only half as sweet as table
sugar, and have the same
amount of kilojoules.
Sweetness relative to table
sugar = 0.55 times less

Maltose
GI 105
16 kJ (4 Calories) per gram
250 kJ (60 Calories) per
teaspoon table sugar
equivalent*

Maltose or malt causes blood
glucose levels to rise rapidly. It
is only one-third as sweet as
table sugar, and has the same
amount of kilojoules.
Sweetness relative to table
sugar = 0.32 times less

Mannitol
GI n/a
9 kJ (2 Calories) per gram
64 kJ (15 Calories) per
teaspoon table sugar
equivalent*
Food additive code 421
(Australia/New Zealand)

Mannitol has no effect
on blood glucose levels.
It is only three-quarters
as sweet as table sugar, but
has only half the amount of
kilojoules, and may have a
laxative effect if eaten in large
quantities.
Sweetness relative to
table sugar = 0.70 times less

Maple syrup
GI 54
11 kJ (3 Calories) per gram
61 kJ (14 Calories) per
teaspoon table sugar
equivalent *

Pure maple syrup has a
moderate effect on blood
glucose levels. It is a little
sweeter than table sugar, but
has less kilojoules.
Sweetness relative to
table sugar = 1.1 times less

Polydextrose
GI 7
5 kJ (1 Calorie) per gram
25 kJ (6 Calories) per
teaspoon table sugar
equivalent*
Food additive code 1200
(Australia/New Zealand)
Also known as Litesse

Polydextrose has very little
effect on blood glucose levels.
It is not sweet, but is used as
a bulking agent with non-
nutritive sweeteners. It has
only one-third the amount of
kilojoules as table sugar, but
may have a laxative effect if
eaten in large quantities.
Sweetness relative to table
sugar = 0

Table sugar (sucrose)
GI 65
16 kJ (4 Calories) per gram
67 kJ (16 Calories) per
teaspoon table sugar
equivalent*
Also known as caster sugar,
brown sugar, raw sugar, icing
sugar

Sucrose or table sugar is the
most common sweetener eaten
in Australia and New Zealand.
Despite popular misconceptions,
when eaten, it causes blood
glucose levels to rise at a
moderate rate.
Sweetness = 1.0

Xylitol
GI 21
12 kJ (3 Calories) per gram
60 kJ (14 Calories) per
teaspoon table sugar
equivalent*
Food additive code 965**

Xylitol is a sugar alcohol that has
essentially no effect on blood
glucose levels. It is as sweet as
sugar and has less kilojoules,
but may have a laxative effect if
consumed in large quantities.
Sweetness relative to table
sugar = 1.0

Non-nutritive sweeteners

Acesulphame potassium or acesulphame K
GI 0
0 kJ (0 Calories) per gram
0 kJ (0 Calories) per teaspoon table sugar equivalent *
Food additive code number 950
Brand names: Sunnett, and found in Hermesetas Gold, Hermesetas with Fructofibres

Acesulphame K is hundreds of times sweeter than sugar, has no effect on blood glucose levels, and doesn't provide any kilojoules because it is not absorbed into the body. Sweetness relative to table sugar = 200 times more

Alitame
GI 0
17 kJ (4 Calories) per gram
0 kJ (0 Calories) per teaspoon table sugar equivalent*
Food additive code number 956**
Brand name: Aclame

Alitame is thousands of times sweeter than sugar, and has essentially no effect on blood glucose levels. Because it is a protein it does provide some kilojoules but because it is so sweet, you only use it in tiny amounts.
Sweetness relative to table sugar = 2000 times more

Aspartame
GI 0
17 kJ (4 Calories) per gram
1.4 kJ (0.3 Calories) per teaspoon table sugar equivalent*
Food additive code number 951**
Brand names: Nutrasweet, Equal, Equal Spoonful, and Sugarless and found in Hermesetas Gold, and Hermesetas with Fructofibres

Aspartame is a couple of hundred times sweeter than sugar, and has essentially no effect on blood glucose levels. Because it is a protein it does provide some kilojoules but because it is very sweet, you only use it in small amounts. Sweetness relative to table sugar = 150–250 times more. *WARNING: Aspartame should not be used by people with phenylketonuria.*

Cyclamate
GI 0
0 kJ (0 Calories) per gram
0 kJ (0 Calories) per teaspoon
table sugar equivalent*
Food additive code number
952**
Brand name: Sucaryl

Cyclamate is tens of times sweeter than sugar, has essentially no effect on blood glucose levels and is not metabolised by most people. Sweetness relative to table sugar = 15–50 times more

Neotame
GI 0
17 kJ (4 Calories) per gram
0 kJ (0 Calories) per teaspoon
table sugar equivalent*
Food additive code number
961**

Neotame is many thousands of times sweeter than sugar, and has essentially no effect on blood glucose levels. Because it is a protein it does provide some kilojoules but because it is extremely sweet, it is only used in tiny amounts. Sweetness relative to table sugar = 7,000–13,000 times more.
While Neotame is a permitted food additive in Australia and New Zealand it is not currently found in any foods or beverages.

Saccharin

GI 0

0 kJ (0 Calories) per gram

0 kJ (0 Calories) per teaspoon table sugar equivalent*

Food additive code number 954**

Brand names: Sugarine, Sugarella, Sweetex, Hermesetas, and Sucaryl

Saccharin is hundreds of times sweeter than sugar, has no effect on blood glucose levels and is not metabolised by the human body. Sweetness relative to table sugar = 300–500 times more

Sucralose

GI 0

0 kJ (0 Calories) per gram

0 kJ (0 Calories) per teaspoon table sugar equivalent teaspoon table sugar equivalent*

Food additive code number 955

Brand name: Splenda

Sucralose is hundreds of times sweeter than sugar, has no effect on blood glucose levels, and does not provide any kilojoules because it is not absorbed into the body. Sweetness relative to table sugar = 400–600 times more

Thaumatin

GI 0

17 kJ (4 Calories) per gram

0 kJ (0 Calories) per teaspoon table sugar equivalent

Food additive code number 957**

Brand name: Talin

Thaumatin is several thousands of times sweeter than sugar, and has essentially no effect on blood glucose levels. Because it is a protein it does provide some kilojoules but because it is so sweet, it is only used in small amounts. Sweetness relative to table sugar = 2,000–3,000 times more

---

* The amount of kilojoules in the volume of alternative sweetener that provides the equivalent sweetness to 1 teaspoon of table sugar.

** Food additive code numbers apply to Australia and New Zealand.

GI values

Using the tables

These tables will help you put low GI food choices into your shopping trolley and on your plate.

Here we give you the best low GI food choices for each category. Each entry lists an individual food and its GI value. We also list the nominal serve size, the amount of carbohydrate per serve, and the GL.

A low GI value is 55 and under
A medium/moderate GI value is 56 to 69 inclusive
A high GI value is 70 or more

You can use the tables to:

❑ Find the GI of your favourite foods
❑ Compare carb-rich foods within a category (two types of bread or breakfast cereal for example)
❑ Identify the best carbohydrate choices
❑ Improve your diet by finding a low GI substitute for high GI foods
❑ Put together a low GI meal
❑ Find foods with a high GI but low GL.

Each individual food appears alphabetically within a food category, like 'Bread' or 'Fruit'. This makes it easy to compare the kinds of foods you eat every day and helps you see which high GI foods you could substitute with low GI versions. If you are unsure of the food category a food might fall under, we've also provided an index to individual foods on pages 206–212.

The food categories used in the tables are:

❑ **Beverages** – including juices and soft drinks

❑ **Biscuits & crackers** – including commercial sweet biscuits, savoury crispbreads and plain crackers

❑ **Breads** – including sliced white and wholemeal bread, fruit breads and flat breads

❑ **Breakfast cereals** – including processed cereals, muesli, oats and porridge

❑ **Dairy products** – including milk, yoghurt, ice-creams and other dairy desserts, and soy products

❑ **Fruit** – including fresh, canned and dried fruit

❑ **Legumes** – including baked beans, chickpeas, lentils and split peas

❑ **Meat, seafood & protein** – including baked beans, chickpeas, lentils and split peas

❑ **Rice, pasta, noodles & grains**

❑ **Snackfoods & treats** – including cakes, chocolate, fruit bars, muesli bars, muffins and nuts

❑ **Spreads & sweeteners** – including sugars, honey and jam

❑ **Takeaway & pre-prepared meals** – including pasta sauces, pre-prepared and convenience foods and soups

❑ **Vegetables** – including green vegetables, salad vegetables, roots and tubers (e.g. potatoes)

❑ **Weight management products** – including meal replacement drinks, bars and soups.

In this version of the tables, the products appear alphabetically within their food category and we have included a household measure for ease of use alongside each entry. We have also included foods that we think have a moderate or high GI but which haven't been tested, using a '●' symbol in place of a GI value. This is to make it clearer which foods have been tested and which haven't. Unfortunately, we can't even make an assumption about the GI value of such foods unless they are very closely related to a food which has been tested. Only more testing will show us the GI value of more foods, so if you want to know the GI value of something you eat and you can't find it here, then contact the manufacturer and suggest they have their food tested.

In the tables you will sometimes see these symbols:

★ indicates that a food contains very little or no carbohydrate which means that the GI isn't relevant (or can't be tested). You will find this symbol beside foods like cheese, fish, chicken, meat and green leafy vegetables. We have included these foods because so many people ask us for their GI.

■ indicates that a food is high in saturated fat.

● indicates that a food does contain carbohydrate but has either not been GI tested or the results of the testing have not been published. To help you manage your blood glucose levels and reduce the

overall GI of your diet you will find this symbol
in these tables besides products like biscuits and
cereals – carb-rich foods that we regularly buy.
Although it's not possible to work out an accurate
GI value for a product based on its ingredients, it is
possible to make an educated guess as to whether
it will be high or low GI, based on similar products
that have been tested.

Ⓖ indicates that a food is part of the GI Symbol
Program. Foods with the GI symbol have had their
GI tested properly and are a healthier choice for
their food category.

All foods have been tested using an internationally
standardised method so you can make a fair comparison.
Gram for gram of carbohydrates, the higher the GI, the
higher the blood glucose levels after consumption. If you
can't find the GI value for a food you regularly eat in these
tables, check out our website (www. glycemicindex.com).
We maintain an international database of published GI
values that have been tested by a reliable laboratory.
Alternatively, please write to the manufacturer and
encourage them to have the food tested by an accredited
laboratory such as the Sydney University Glycemic Index
Research Service (SUGiRS). In the meantime, choose a
similar food from the tables as a substitute.

Category index

BEVERAGES

FOOD	GI	SAMPLE SERVING	AVAILABLE CARB (g) PER SERVE	GL PER SERVE
Alcohol				
Beer, Tooheys New Draught (4.6% alcohol)	66	I bottle, 375ml	12	8
Fruit juices				
Apple juice, Berri	39	200ml	21	8
Apple juice, no added sugar	40	I cup, 250ml	28	11
Apple juice, filtered, Wild About Fruit	44	I cup, 250ml	30	13
Apple juice, pure, Granny Smith	44	I cup, 250ml	30	13
Apple juice, Wild About Fruit	37	I cup, 250ml	28	10
Apple & Blackcurrant juice, Berri	43	200ml	21	9
Apple & Cherry juice, Wild About Fruit	43	I cup, 250ml	33	14
Apple & Mango juice, Wild About Fruit	47	I cup, 250ml	34	16
Apple, Pine, Passion juice, Wild About Fruit	48	I cup, 250ml	33	16

★ little or no carbs ■ high in saturated fat ● untested/unknown © GI Symbol partner
Low GI = less than or equal to 55

BEVERAGES

FOOD	GI	SAMPLE SERVING	AVAILABLE CARB (g) PER SERVE	GL PER SERVE
Fruit juices (continued)				
Australian Grown – Berri juice				
Apple juice (no added sugar)	45	200ml	21	10
Apple, Mango juice (no added sugar)	48	200ml	24	12
Apple, Passionfruit juice (no added sugar)	48	200ml	24	11
Apple, Mango, Banana juice (no added sugar)	46	200ml	22	10
Apple, Pear juice	45	200ml	22	10
Apple, Pear & Mango juice	47	200ml	23	11
Apple, Pear & Passionfruit juice	42	200ml	22	9
Apple, Pineapple juice (no added sugar)	45	200ml	21	10
Apple, Pineapple, Guava juice	51	200ml	22	11
Apple, Strawberry juice (no added sugar)	48	200ml	26	12
Breakfast juice (no added sugar)	46	200ml	21	10

★ little or no carbs   ■ high in saturated fat   ● untested/unknown   ☺ GI Symbol partner
Low GI = less than or equal to 55

BEVERAGES

FOOD	GI	SAMPLE SERVING	AVAILABLE CARB (g) PER SERVE	GL PER SERVE
Fruit juices (continued)				
Orange juice, low acid	37	200ml	17	6
Orange & Mango juice	46	200ml	22	10
Orange juice, pulp free	37	200ml	17	6
Orange juice (no added sugar)	37	200ml	17	6
Pineapple, Orange & Mango juice	53	200ml	20	11
Carrot juice, freshly made	43	1 cup, 250ml	14	6
Apricot Nectar 25%, Berri Classics	65	200ml	27	18
Coconut water, Nudie	55	1 bottle, 350ml	18	10
Cranberry Fruit Drink 25%, Berri Classics	65	200ml	26	17
Cranberry Juice Cocktail, Ocean Spray	52	1 cup, 250ml	31	16
Five Fruits juice, Daily Juice	49	200ml	20	10
Grape juice, Berri Classics	49	200ml	28	14
Grapefruit juice, Berri	49	1 cup, 250ml	18	9

★ little or no carbs ■ high in saturated fat ● untested/unknown © GI Symbol partner
Low GI = less than or equal to 55

BEVERAGES

FOOD	GI	SAMPLE SERVING	AVAILABLE CARB (g) PER SERVE	GL PER SERVE
Fruit juices (continued)				
Grapefruit juice, unsweetened	48	1 cup, 250ml	20	10
Multi-V juice, Berri (no added sugar)	46	200ml	21	9
Orange juice, Berri (no added sugar)	49	200ml	18	9
Orange juice, fresh, unsweetened	50	1 cup, 250ml	18	9
Orange juice, unsweetened, from concentrate, Quelch	53	1 cup, 250ml	18	10
Orange & Mango juice, Daily Juice	48	200ml	21	10
Pineapple juice, Berri (no added sugar)	49	200ml	19	9
Pineapple juice, unsweetened	46	1 cup, 250ml	34	16
Pomegranate juice, POM Wonderful	53	1 cup, 250ml	34	18
Prune juice, Golden Circle Healthy Life Natural	43	1 cup, 250ml	38	16
Super Juice Immune juice, Berri	47	200ml	22	10
Tomato juice	38	1 cup, 250ml	14	5

★ little or no carbs ■ high in saturated fat ● untested/unknown ☺ GI Symbol partner
Low GI = less than or equal to 55

BEVERAGES

FOOD	GI	SAMPLE SERVING	AVAILABLE CARB (g) PER SERVE	GL PER SERVE
Fruit juices (continued)				
Tomato juice, no added sugar, Berri	41	200ml	8	3
Vegetable juice	43	1 cup, 250ml	9	4
Ribena blackcurrant fruit syrup, reconstituted	52	1 cup, 250ml	32	17
Coles				
© Apple Blackcurrant NAS	43	200ml	21	9
© Apple NAS	45	200ml	21	10
© Multi Vit Juice NAS	46	200ml	21	9
© Orange Mango Juice NAS	46	200ml	22	10
© Orange NAS	49	200ml	18	9
© Pineapple Juice	49	200ml	19	9
© Tomato Juice	41	200ml	8	3
Milkshakes, smoothies & sports drinks (see also Dairy Products)				
AdVital nutritionally complete powdered supplement	48	40g	20	10

★ little or no carbs ■ high in saturated fat ● untested/unknown © GI Symbol partner
Low GI = less than or equal to 55

BEVERAGES

FOOD	GI	SAMPLE SERVING	AVAILABLE CARB (g) PER SERVE	GL PER SERVE

Milkshakes, smoothies & sports drinks (continued) (see also Dairy Products)

FOOD	GI	SAMPLE SERVING	AVAILABLE CARB (g) PER SERVE	GL PER SERVE
Aussie Bodies Start the Day UHT.				
Choc Banana flavoured drink	24	1 cup, 250ml	15	4
Chocolate flavoured drink	26	1 cup, 250ml	15	4
Aussie Bodies Trim Protein Shake				
Chocolate flavoured	39	1 cup, 250ml	12	5
French Vanilla flavoured	41	1 cup, 250ml	12	5
Blackmores				
Superfruit Smoothie Meal				
Replacement Creamy Vanilla	17	45g dry powder	18	3
Dark Chocolate &				
Blackcurrant	21	45g dry powder	17	4
Mixed Berries	23	45g dry powder	18	4
Build-Up, drink powder, vanilla				
with fibre, in water, Nestlé	41	1 cup, 250ml	35	14
Chocolate Hazelnut				
soy smoothie	34	1 cup, 250ml	25	8
Ⓖ Complete Hot Chocolate mix				
made with hot water, Nestlé	51	1 cup, 250ml	23	12
Devondale Fast Start varieties				
Chocolate Liquid Breakfast	39	250ml	30	12
Coffee Liquid Breakfast	39	250ml	31	12
Vanilla Liquid Breakfast	39	250ml	30	12

★ little or no carbs ■ high in saturated fat ● untested/unknown Ⓖ GI Symbol partner
Low GI = less than or equal to 55

BEVERAGES

FOOD	GI	SAMPLE SERVING	AVAILABLE CARB (g) PER SERVE	GL PER SERVE
Milkshakes, smoothies & sports drinks (continued) (see also Dairy Products)				
Ensure, vanilla drink	48	1 cup, 250ml	34	16
Gatorade	78	1 cup, 250ml	15	12
Hi-Pro energy drink mix, vanilla, Harrod foods, mixed in reduced-fat milk	36	1 cup, 250ml	19	7
Isostar	70	1 cup, 250ml	18	13
iSustain Hospital Quality Vanilla flavour powdered beverage	37	60g	38	14
iSustain Hospital Quality Vanilla flavour plus Fibre powdered beverage	35	60g	34	12
iSustain Hospital Quality Chocolate flavour plus Fibre powdered beverage	33	60g	33	11
Jevity, fibre-enriched drink	48	1 can, 237ml	36	17
Kellogg's Coco Pops Chocolatey Liquid Breakfast	35	250ml	25	9
Kellogg's Nutri-Grain Breakfast Fuel	38	250ml	23	9

★ little or no carbs ■ high in saturated fat ● untested/unknown ☺ GI Symbol partner
Low GI = less than or equal to 55

BEVERAGES

FOOD	GI	SAMPLE SERVING	AVAILABLE CARB (g) PER SERVE	GL PER SERVE

Milkshakes, smoothies & sports drinks (continued) (see also Dairy Products)

FOOD	GI	SAMPLE SERVING	AVAILABLE CARB (g) PER SERVE	GL PER SERVE
LEAN Nutrimeal drink powder, Dutch Chocolate	26	1 cup, 250ml	13	3
Lucozade, original, sparkling glucose drink	95	1 cup, 250ml	42	40
☺ Nestlé Milo Ready-to-drink	34	200ml	22	7
☺ Nutrimeal meal replacement drink, Usana (all flavours)	25	1 cup, 250ml	17	3
☺ Nutrimeal Free meal replacement drink, Usana	49	290ml	27	13
Proform Hi-protein powder, neutral flavour, prepared with skim milk, MGC Dairy Co.	45	1 cup, 250ml	49	22
Proform Hi-protein powder, vanilla flavour, prepared with skim milk, MGC Dairy Co.	42	1 cup, 250ml	50	21
ReduceXS Chocolate Deluxe formulated meal replacement powder, prepared with water	10	1 cup, 250ml	8	1

★ little or no carbs ■ high in saturated fat ● untested/unknown ☺ GI Symbol partner
Low GI = less than or equal to 55

BEVERAGES

FOOD	GI	SAMPLE SERVING	AVAILABLE CARB (g) PER SERVE	GL PER SERVE
Milkshakes, smoothies & sports drinks (continued) (see also Dairy Products)				
Sanitarium Up & Go varieties				
Vanilla Ice	22	250ml	30	7
Banana	27	250ml	30	8
Choc Ice	34	250ml	30	10
Energize Coffee	35	350ml	34	12
Energize Vanilla	38	350ml	34	13
Energize Chocolate	33	350ml	37	12
Sustagen varieties				
© Diabetic Vanilla (powder)	34	55g	25	8
© Diabetic Vanilla (liquid)	30	1 tetrapack, 237ml	23	7
© Everyday Formula Dutch Choc	36	15g	11	4
© Everyday Formula Vanilla	36	15g	11	4
© Hospital Formula Chocolate	44	60g	39	17
© Hospital Formula Neutral	46	60g	39	18
Hospital Formula Vanilla	44	60g	39	17
© Hospital Formula Plus Fibre, Chocolate	33	60g	39	13
© Hospital Formula Plus Fibre, Vanilla	33	60g	39	13
© Instant pudding	27	57g	34	9
© Optimum	49	55g	29	14
© Ready-to-drink Vanilla	39	250ml	42	16
© Ready-to-drink Chocolate	50	250ml	42	21
© Sports drink, Chocolate	43	60g	39	17
© Sports drink, Vanilla	43	60g	39	17

★ little or no carbs ■ high in saturated fat ● untested/unknown © GI Symbol partner
Low GI = less than or equal to 55

BEVERAGES

FOOD	GI	SAMPLE SERVING	AVAILABLE CARB (g) PER SERVE	GL PER SERVE
Milkshakes, smoothies & sports drinks (continued) (see also Dairy Products)				
Tony Ferguson's Meal Replacement Shake, all flavours, prepared with water	22	I cup, 250ml	28	6
Soft drinks				
Coca-Cola	53	I can, 375ml	40	21
Cordial, orange, reconstituted	66	I cup, 250ml	20	13
Fanta	68	I can, 375ml	51	35
Lemonade, Schweppes	54	I can, 375ml	42	23
Solo, lemon squash	58	I can, 375ml	44	26
Tropical blend fruit drink	47	I cup, 250ml	28	13

★ little or no carbs ■ high in saturated fat ● untested/unknown © GI Symbol partner
Low GI = less than or equal to 55

BISCUITS & CRACKERS

FOOD	GI	SAMPLE SERVING	AVAILABLE CARB (g) PER SERVE	GL PER SERVE
Sweet biscuits				
Generic				
Chocolate chip cookies (made with coconut flour)	43■	2 biscuits, 20g	16	7
Coconut macaroons	32	2 biscuits, 20g	1	4
Oatmeal, Highland	55	2 biscuits, 20g	14	8
Oatmeal	54	2 biscuits, 20g	14	8
Rich tea	55	2 biscuits, 20g	13	7
Shortbread, plain	64■	2 biscuits, 25g	16	10
Vanilla wafer, cream-filled	77■	3 biscuits, 25g	18	14
Arnott's				
Full o' Fruit	●	2 biscuits, 20g	15	●
Ginger Nut	●	1 biscuit, 13g	11	●
Kingston	48	1 biscuit, 13g	8	4
Malt-O-Milk	●	3 biscuits, 21g	16	●
Marie	●	2 biscuits, 16g	12	●

★ little or no carbs ■ high in saturated fat ● untested/unknown ⓒ GI Symbol partner
Low GI = less than or equal to 55

BISCUITS & CRACKERS

FOOD	GI	SAMPLE SERVING	AVAILABLE CARB (g) PER SERVE	GL PER SERVE
Sweet biscuits (continued)				
Arnott's continued				
Milk Arrowroot	69	2 biscuits, 16g	12	8
Morning Coffee	79	3 biscuits, 17g	12	9
Shredded Wheatmeal	62	3 biscuits, 23g	15	9
Snack Right varieties (apple & sultana, wild berry, fruit pillow)	45–52	2 biscuits, 33g	24	12
Snack Right sultana, fruit slice	48	2 biscuits, 20g	22	11
Snack Right sultana, choc fruit slice	45	2 biscuits, 25g	17	8
Spicy Fruit Roll	●	1 biscuit, 17g	12	●
Tic Toc	●	2 biscuits, 18g	13	●
Carman's				
Carman's Apricot and Almond Rounds	46	1 serve, 40g	22	10
Carman's Classic Fruit Muesli Rounds	42	1 serve, 40g	22	9

★ little or no carbs ■ high in saturated fat ● untested/unknown ⊚ GI Symbol partner
Low GI = less than or equal to 55

BISCUITS & CRACKERS

FOOD	GI	SAMPLE SERVING	AVAILABLE CARB (g) PER SERVE	GL PER SERVE
Sweet biscuits (continued)				
Griffin's				
Fruitli Golden Fruit	77	2 biscuits, 25g	17	13
Maltmeal Wafer	50	2 biscuits, 25g	17	9
Paradise				
Vive Lites, caramel pecan	●	2 biscuits, 21g	16	●
Vive Lites, choc chip mini cookies	●	1 mini pack, 30g	24	●
Vive Wellbeing, date & ginger	●	2 biscuits, 18g	13	●
Weight Watchers				
Butternut	●	2 biscuits, 18g	14	●
Fruit Slice	●	2 cookies, 23g	17	●
Triple Choc	●	2 biscuits, 18g	11	●
Savoury biscuits				
Generic				
Rice cake, puffed	82	2 slices, 20g	15	12
Rice cracker	91	12 crackers, 20g	16	15

★ little or no carbs ■ high in saturated fat ● untested/unknown ⓖ GI Symbol partner
Low GI = less than or equal to 55

BISCUITS & CRACKERS

FOOD	GI	SAMPLE SERVING	AVAILABLE CARB (g) PER SERVE	GL PER SERVE
Savoury biscuits (continued)				
Arnott's				
Breton	67■	6 crackers, 26g	15	10
Cruskits varieties				
Corn	●	4 crackers, 19g	14	●
Light	●	4 crackers, 23g	17	●
Rye	●	4 crackers, 19g	12	●
Jatz	55■	6 crackers, 25g	13	7
Jatz 97% fat free	●	5 crackers, 19g	15	●
Salada varieties				
Light original	●	1 cracker, 14g	11	●
Light poppy & sesame	●	1 cracker, 14g	11	●
Multigrain 97% fat free	●	1 cracker, 14g	11	●
Original	●	1 cracker, 14g	10	●
Wholemeal	●	1 cracker, 14g	9	●
Sao	70	3 crackers, 26g	16	11
Shapes, barbecue	48	10 crackers, 23g	15	7
Thin Captain	●	3 crackers, 17g	12	●

★ little or no carbs   ■ high in saturated fat   ● untested/unknown   © GI Symbol partner
Low GI = less than or equal to 55

BISCUITS & CRACKERS

FOOD	GI	SAMPLE SERVING	AVAILABLE CARB (g) PER SERVE	GL PER SERVE
Savoury biscuits (continued)				
Vita-Weat varieties				
9-Grain	●	2 sandwich, 23g	15	●
9-Grain	●	4 regular, 25g	14	●
Cracked Pepper	●	4 regular, 23g	16	●
Grain Snacks, all varieties	●	1 packet, 20g	13	●
Lunch Slices Soy, Linseed & Sesame	52	2 crispbread, 38g	22	11
Lunch Slices, Sunflower, Pumpkin & Canola	59	2 crispbread, 38g	22	13
Original	●	4 regular, 25g	16	●
Sesame	●	4 regular, 23g	13	●
Soy & Linseed	●	4 regular, 23g	13	●
Paradise				
Vive Lites Wholemeal crispbread	●	4 biscuits, 28g	20	●
Vive Wellbeing 7 Grains crispbread	●	4 biscuits, 32g	20	●
Ryvita varieties				
Pumpkin Seeds & Oats crispbread	46	2 slices, 25g	14	6
Sunflower Seeds & Oats crispbread	48	2 slices, 25g	14	7

★ little or no carbs ■ high in saturated fat ● untested/unknown ⊙ GI Symbol partner
Low GI = less than or equal to 55

BISCUITS & CRACKERS

FOOD	GI	SAMPLE SERVING	AVAILABLE CARB (g) PER SERVE	GL PER SERVE
Savoury biscuits (continued)				
Water Cracker	78	6 crackers, 18g	14	11
Corn Thins, puffed corn, Real Foods	87	4 slices, 23g	16	14
Kavli Norwegian crispbread	71	4 thins, 20g	13	9

★ little or no carbs ■ high in saturated fat ● untested/unknown ⓒ GI Symbol partner
Low GI = less than or equal to 55

BREADS

FOOD	GI	SAMPLE SERVING	AVAILABLE CARB (g) PER SERVE	GL PER SERVE
Bread & bakery products				
Bakers Delight				
Apricot Delight				
log	56	1 slice, 43g	24	13
roll	56	1 roll, 80g	48	27
scroll	56	1 scroll, 105g	60	34
Authentic sourdough				
loaf	58	1 toast slice, 33g	16	9
roll	58	1 roll, 115g	59	34
Block loaf, wholemeal	71	1 toast slice, 38g	14	10
Cape Seed				
loaf	48	1 toast slice, 45g	13	6
roll	48	1 roll, 89g	27	13
Cape Fruit & Nut roll	55	1 roll, 89g	33	18
Chia, white	63	1 toast slice, 40g	17	11
Country Grain loaf	61	1 toast slice, 38g	19	12
Soy & Linseed loaf	59	1 toast slice, 48g	14	8
Tiger loaf, white	71	1 toast slice, 37g	17	12
Toasty Fruit loaf	61	1 toast slice, 37g	25	15

★ little or no carbs ■ high in saturated fat ● untested/unknown Ⓖ GI Symbol partner
Low GI = less than or equal to 55

BREADS

FOOD	GI	SAMPLE SERVING	AVAILABLE CARB (g) PER SERVE	GL PER SERVE
Bread & bakery products (continued)				
Wholemeal Country Grain				
block loaf	53	1 toast slice, 40g	15	8
dinner roll	53	1 roll, 34g	13	7
long roll	53	1 roll, 65g	27	14
round roll	53	1 roll, 65g	27	14
Bill's Organic Breads				
Sourdough Multigrain	●	1 slice, 35g	15	●
Bürgen				
ⓖ Fruit & Muesli	53	1 slice, 42g	19	10
ⓖ Pumpkin Seeds	51	1 slice, 42g	11	6
ⓖ Rye	53	1 slice, 42g	14	7
ⓖ Soy-Lin	52	1 slice, 42g	13	7
ⓖ Wholegrains & Oats	51	1 slice, 42g	13	7
ⓖ Wholemeal & Seeds	39	1 slice, 42g	9	4
Buttercup				
Mighty Soft raisin toast	60	1 slice, 35g	20	12
Coles				
ⓖ In-store bakery, 7 seeds & grains	45	2 slices, 70g	22	10
ⓖ In-store bakery, low GI Harvest Grain bread	51	2 slices, 70g	38	19

★ little or no carbs   ■ high in saturated fat   ● untested/unknown   ⓖ GI Symbol partner
Low GI = less than or equal to 55

BREADS

FOOD	GI	SAMPLE SERVING	AVAILABLE CARB (g) PER SERVE	GL PER SERVE
Bread & bakery products (continued)				
⊚ In-store bakery, high fibre low GI white bread	55	2 slices, 80g	31	17
Country Life Bakery				
Low GI white	54	2 slices, 78g	29	16
Diego's				
White corn tortillas	53	1 regular, 56g	27	14
Reduced carb wraps	51	1 regular, 43g	11	6
Golden Hearth				
Heavy Wholegrain Organic	53	1 large slice, 50g	21	11
Helga's				
Lower Carb 5 Seeds bread	53	2 slices, 70g	19	10
Lower Carb Soy & Toasted Sesame bread	51	2 slices, 70g	20	10
Mixed Grain Wrap	55	1 wrap, 70g	33	18
Herman Brot				
Low Carb bread	24	1 slice, 45g	2	1
Lawson's				
Settlers' Grain	65	2 slices, 114g	47	7

★ little or no carbs ■ high in saturated fat ● untested/unknown ⊚ GI Symbol partner
Low GI = less than or equal to 55

BREADS

FOOD	GI	SAMPLE SERVING	AVAILABLE CARB (g) PER SERVE	GL PER SERVE
Bread & bakery products (continued)				
Mission Foods				
Chia Wraps	50	I wrap, 48g	19	9
Red Quinoa Wraps	59	I wrap, 48g	20	12
ⓒ White corn tortillas	52	I wrap, 26g	11	6
Molenberg				
12 Grains & Seeds Original bread	67	I slice, 37g	16	11
12 Grains & Seeds Soy & Linseed bread	64	I slice, 37g	14	9
Naturis				
Gluten-free, buckwheat	72	I slice, 48g	17	12
New Freedom Bakery				
Farmhouse White Loaf	50	I slice, 42g	16	8
Old El Paso				
Whole Grain Tortillas (2× Fibre)	50	I tortilla, 40g	19	9

★ little or no carbs ■ high in saturated fat ● untested/unknown ⓒ GI Symbol partner
Low GI = less than or equal to 55

BREADS

FOOD	GI	SAMPLE SERVING	AVAILABLE CARB (g) PER SERVE	GL PER SERVE
Bread & bakery products (continued)				
Pav's Bakery				
Spelt Multigrain	54	1 slice, 30g	12	7
Tip Top				
Café hot cross buns	59	1 bun, 88g	49	29
© 9-Grain Original	53	1 slice, 37g	13	7
© 9-Grain Pumpkin Seed	52	1 slice, 37g	13	7
© 9-Grain Wholemeal	53	1 slice, 38g	12	6
Raisin toast, Retreats	63	1 slice, 33g	19	12
Spicy Fruit loaf	54	1 slice, 36g	19	10
Sunblest, white	71	1 slice, 30g	14	10
Sunblest, wholemeal	71	1 slice, 30g	12	9
Wonder White				
Hi Fibre Plus white bread	74	1 slice, 35g	14	10
Wholemeal Smooth Wholemeal & Iron bread	73	1 slice, 35g	14	10
Vitamins & Minerals white bread	76	1 slice, 35g	15	11

★ little or no carbs ■ high in saturated fat ● untested/unknown © GI Symbol partner
Low GI = less than or equal to 55

BREADS

FOOD	GI	SAMPLE SERVING	AVAILABLE CARB (g) PER SERVE	GL PER SERVE
Bread & bakery products (continued)				
Woolworth's Select				
Traditional white corn tortilla	53	1 regular, 56g	27	14
Reduced carb tortilla	51	1 regular, 43g	16	8
Specialty breads & baked foods				
Bagel	72	1 large, 85g	43	31
Baguette, traditional French	77	¼ loaf, 62g	33	25
Breadcrumbs, white	●	¼ loaf, 30g	20	●
Chapatti, corn	59	1 small, 35g	14	8
Chapatti, bajra	49	1 small, 35g	14	7
Chapatti, barley	48	1 small, 35g	14	8
Continental fruit	47	1 thick slice, 45g	24	11
Croissant	67	1 large, 70g	24	16
Croissant, All Butter, Coles	46	1 croissant, 63g	26	12
Crumpet, white	69	1 regular, 50g	16	11

★ little or no carbs ■ high in saturated fat ● untested/unknown © GI Symbol partner
Low GI = less than or equal to 55

BREADS

FOOD	GI	SAMPLE SERVING	AVAILABLE CARB (g) PER SERVE	GL PER SERVE
Specialty breads & baked foods (continued)				
Doughnut, commercial, cinnamon	75	1 regular, 50g	25	30
English muffin	77	1 regular, 64g	23	18
Foccacia	●	1 piece, 50g	21	●
Fruit bun, iced	●	1 regular, 85g	39	●
Gluten-free bread, commercial	●	1 medium slice, 30g	16	●
Hamburger bun	61	1 regular, 90g	45	27
Hotdog bun, white	68	1 regular, 62g	33	22
Hot cross bun, choc chip	●	1 regular, 65g	41	●
Hot cross bun, homemade	66	1 regular, 70g	31	21
Italian bread	73	1 slice, 40g	18	13
Italian breadsticks, grissini	●	3 sticks, 25g	18	●
Lavash, white	●	1 piece, 67g	36	●
Lavash, wholemeal	●	1 piece, 67g	33	●

★ little or no carbs ■ high in saturated fat ● untested/unknown © GI Symbol partner
Low GI = less than or equal to 55

BREADS

FOOD	GI	SAMPLE SERVING	AVAILABLE CARB (g) PER SERVE	GL PER SERVE
Specialty breads & baked foods (continued)				
Kaiser roll, white	73	1 regular, 108g	60	44
Lebanese bread, wholemeal	●	1 large, 100g	48	●
Lebanese bread, white, Seda Bakery	75	1 large, 100g	53	40
Matzo, Jewish bread	●	1 piece, 30g	24	●
Melba toast, plain	70	30g	23	16
Middle Eastern flatbread	91	30g	17	16
Wrap, Mountain Bread Oat	62	1 piece 25g	13	8
Multigrain bread	65	1 slice, 34g	15	10
Naan, traditional, True Foods	71	1 small naan, 63g	27	19
Pancakes, buckwheat, gluten-free, packet mix, Orgran	102	1/10 pkt, 37g	29	30
Pancakes, gluten-free, packet mix, Freedom Foods	61	1 serve, 80g	53	32
Pancakes, homemade	●	1 regular, 56g	16	●
Pancakes, shaker mix, Green's	67	1 regular, 50g	23	15

★ little or no carbs ■ high in saturated fat ● untested/unknown ⊚ GI Symbol partner
Low GI = less than or equal to 55

122

BREADS

FOOD	GI	SAMPLE SERVING	AVAILABLE CARB (g) PER SERVE	GL PER SERVE
Specialty breads & baked foods (continued)				
Pappadum, microwaved	●	4 regular, 24g	11	●
Pikelets, commercial, Golden	85	1 regular, 25g	9	8
Pikelets, shake mix	●	1 regular, 35g	16	●
Pita bread, white	57	1 regular, 60g	33	19
Pizza base, Boboli Original Crust	52	50g	24	12
Pumpernickel bread	50	1 slice, 47g	21	11
Roll, white	71	1 regular, 65g	34	24
Roll, white, dinner	71	1 small, 30g	16	11
Roll, wholemeal	70	1 regular, 65g	26	18
Roll, cheese & bacon	●	1 regular, 75g	27	●
Rye bread, light	68	1 slice, 30g	14	10
Rye bread, dark	76	1 slice, 30g	13	10
Rye bread, wholemeal	58	1 slice, 30g	13	8
Scone, plain, packet mix, Defiance	92	1 regular, 40g	16	15
Scone, fruit	●	1 regular, 40g	22	●

★ little or no carbs ■ high in saturated fat ● untested/unknown ⓒ GI Symbol partner
Low GI = less than or equal to 55

BREADS

FOOD	GI	SAMPLE SERVING	AVAILABLE CARB (g) PER SERVE	GL PER SERVE
Specialty breads & baked foods (continued)				
Sliced bread, white	71	1 slice, 32g	14	10
Sliced bread, wholemeal	71	1 slice, 32g	12	9
Sourdough, wheat	54	1 large slice, 64g	33	18
Sourdough, rye	48	1 large slice, 64g	28	13
Stuffing, bread	74	100g	22	16
Taco shell, corn	68	1 large, 20g	11	7
Turkish pide	87	1 small roll, 85g	40	35
Waffles, plain	76	1 regular, 33g	19	14

★ little or no carbs ■ high in saturated fat ● untested/unknown ⓒ GI Symbol partner
Low GI = less than or equal to 55

BREAKFAST CEREALS

FOOD	GI	SAMPLE SERVING	AVAILABLE CARB (g) PER SERVE	GL PER SERVE
Generic				
Buckwheat, puffed	65	14g	12	8
Natural muesli	40	½ cup, 45g	27	11
Oat Bran, raw, unprocessed	55	⅓ cup, 30g	15	8
Porridge, regular oats with water	58	1 cup, 260g	21	12
Porridge, steel-cut oats with water	52	¾ cup, 170g	17	9
Rice Bran, extruded	19	⅓ cup, 30g	14	3
Rice porridge	88	100g	9	8
Semolina, cooked	55	1 cup, 245g	17	9
Shredded wheat	75	1 biscuit, 24g	16	12
Traditional rolled oats	57	30g	18	10
Wheat flake biscuit	69	1 biscuit, 15g	10	7
BelVita Breakfast Biscuits				
Cranberry	40	4 biscuits, 50g	34	14
Crunchy Oats	54	4 biscuits, 50g	34	18
Fruit & Fibre	47	4 biscuits, 50g	34	15

★ little or no carbs ■ high in saturated fat ● untested/unknown © GI Symbol partner
Low GI = less than or equal to 55

BREAKFAST CEREALS

FOOD	GI	SAMPLE SERVING	AVAILABLE CARB (g) PER SERVE	GL PER SERVE
Honey & Nut with Choc Chips	46	4 biscuits, 50g	34	16
Milk and Cereals	45	4 biscuits, 50g	36	16
Be Natural				
Cashew, Almond, Hazelnut & Coconut Muesli	54	¾ cup, 45g	27	15
Multi-Grain Porridge	50	I sachet, 40g	22	11
Pink Lady Apple & Flame Raisin Muesli	51	¾ cup, 45g	31	16
Carman's				
Classic Fruit & Nut Muesli	50	45g	23	12
Cranberry, Apple & Roasted Nut Crunchy Clusters	54	45g	27	15
Deluxe Gluten-free Muesli	49	35g	22	11
Fruit & Seed Porridge	64	40g serve prepared with water	23	15
Honey Roasted Nut Porridge	66	40g serve prepared with water	21	14
Honey Roasted Nut Crunchy Clusters	51	45g	24	12

★ little or no carbs ■ high in saturated fat ● untested/unknown ⊛ GI Symbol partner
Low GI = less than or equal to 55

BREAKFAST CEREALS

FOOD	GI	SAMPLE SERVING	AVAILABLE CARB (g) PER SERVE	GL PER SERVE
Natural Bircher Muesli	48	45g	23	11
Original Fruit-Free Muesli	45	45g	23	10
Super Berry Cranberry, Blueberry & Goji Muesli	41	45g	21	8
Traditional Australian Super Oats, made with water	60	45g serve prepared with water	28	17
Coles				
@ Apricot, Almond & Date Muesli	44	50g	24	11
Smart Buy Muesli	46	50g	29	14
@ Summer Fruits Muesli	54	50g	26	14
@ Vanilla Flavoured Oat Clusters	54	45g	28	15
Freedom Foods				
FreeOats Crunchola, Apple & Blueberry	54	66g	44	24
FreeOats Crunchola, Apple & Cinnamon	52	66g	43	22
FreeOats Crunchola, Berries & Vanilla	47	66g	45	21
Gluten-free muesli	39	40g	13	5

★ little or no carbs ■ high in saturated fat ● untested/unknown @ GI Symbol partner
Low GI = less than or equal to 55

BREAKFAST CEREALS

FOOD	GI	SAMPLE SERVING	AVAILABLE CARB (g) PER SERVE	GL PER SERVE
Hi-Lite	54	100g	68	37
Quick Oats porridge	●	100g	62	●
Yeast-free muesli	44	40g	13	6
Goodness Superfoods				
Digestive 1st	39	45g	21	8
FibreBoost Sprinkles	34	30g	19	6
Heart 1st	46	45g	20	9
Protein 1st	36	45g	17	6
Quick Sachets Barley + Oats 1st: Apple & Honey Porridge	55	35g serve prepared with water	25	14
Traditional Barley + Oats 1st: Porridge	47	40g serve prepared with water	25	12
Kellogg's				
All-Bran Original	55	¾ cup, 45g	20	11
All-Bran varieties				
Wheat Flakes	59	⅔ cup, 30g	21	12
Honey Almond	55	½ cup, 45g	27	15
Apple Flavoured Crunch	57	½ cup, 45g	29	17

★ little or no carbs ■ high in saturated fat ● untested/unknown ☺ GI Symbol partner
Low GI = less than or equal to 55

BREAKFAST CEREALS

FOOD	GI	SAMPLE SERVING	AVAILABLE CARB (g) PER SERVE	GL PER SERVE
All-Bran varieties (continued)				
High Fibre Muesli: Almond & Apricot with Sultanas and Pepita	54	45g	24	13
High Fibre Muesli: Cranberry & Pink Lady Apple with Pepita	49	45g	25	12
Corn Flakes	77	1 cup, 30g	25	19
Crispix	87	1 cup, 30g	26	23
Crunchy Nut varieties				
Corn Flakes	72	⅔ cup, 30g	25	18
Clusters	●	⅓ cup, 30g	23	●
Froot Loops	69	¾ cup, 30g	26	18
Frosties	55	¾ cup, 30g	27	15
Guardian	34	⅔ cup, 30g	19	6
Just Right Original	60	¾ cup, 45g	32	19
Mini-Wheats varieties				
Blackcurrant	72	⅔ cup, 40g	28	20
5 Grains, no fruit filling	58	¾ cup, 40g	27	16
Nutri-Grain Breakfast Fuel	38	1 cup, 30g	23	9
Rice Bubbles	87	1 cup, 30g	26	23

★ little or no carbs   ■ high in saturated fat   ● untested/unknown   ⓒ GI Symbol partner
Low GI = less than or equal to 55

BREAKFAST CEREALS

FOOD	GI	SAMPLE SERVING	AVAILABLE CARB (g) PER SERVE	GL PER SERVE
Special K Original	53	¾ cup, 30g	21	11
Special K varieties				
Advantage	●	1 cup, 40g	26	●
Forest Berries	●	¾ cup, 30g	21	●
Fruit & Nut Medley	55	¾ cup, 40g	26	14
Honey Almond	●	⅔ cup, 30g	22	●
Sultana Bran varieties				
Crunch	●	⅔ cup, 45g	32	●
Original	64	¾ cup, 45g	29	18
Lowan				
Fusion muesli, all varieties	●	45g	26–28	●
Muesli, all varieties	●	45g	26–28	●
Quick Oats	●	30g	18	●
Rolled Oats	59	½ cup, 50g	31	18
Monster Muesli				
Multi-Grain porridge	55	60g	35	19
Morning Sun				
☺ Apricot & Almond muesli	49	45g	26	13
97% Fat-Free Fruit muesli	49	45g	30	15

★ little or no carbs   ■ high in saturated fat   ● untested/unknown   ☺ GI Symbol partner
Low GI = less than or equal to 55

BREAKFAST CEREALS

FOOD	GI	SAMPLE SERVING	AVAILABLE CARB (g) PER SERVE	GL PER SERVE
© Nuts & Seeds fruit-free muesli	55	⅔ cup, 60g	30	17
© Peach & Pecan muesli	49	45g	26	13
Nestlé				
© Milo Protein Clusters	47	45g	28	13
Sanitarium				
Granola Clusters, all varieties	●	50g	35	●
Honey Weets	●	30g	24	●
Light 'n' Tasty, all varieties	68	40g	27–29	19
Natural muesli	49	30g	19	10
Puffed Wheat	80	30g	21	17
Skippy corn flakes	93	30g	24	22
Weet-Bix varieties				
Bites, all varieties	●	45g	30–34	●
Energise	●	2 biscuits, 50g	30	●
Hi-Bran	61	2 biscuits, 40g	22	13
Kids	●	1 biscuit, 15g	10	●
Multigrain	●	1 biscuit, 24g	17	●
Organic	●	2 biscuits, 30g	20	●
Original	69	2 biscuits, 33g	22	15

★ little or no carbs ■ high in saturated fat ● untested/unknown © GI Symbol partner
Low GI = less than or equal to 55

BREAKFAST CEREALS

FOOD	GI	SAMPLE SERVING	AVAILABLE CARB (g) PER SERVE	GL PER SERVE
Uncle Tobys				
Bran Plus	●	45g	12	●
Cheerios	●	30g	22	●
Healthwise Heart Wellbeing	●	45g	29	●
Muesli, Original Swiss Style	62	30g	18	11
Oat Brits	●	42g	26	●
O&G Crunchy Granola Protein Almond & Vanilla	48	45g	28	13
O&G Crunchy Granola Protein Cranberry, Hazelnut & Pepita	52	45g	28	15
Plus varieties Fibre Lift	●	45g	29	●
Protein Lift	●	45g	33	●
Sports Lift	●	45g	32	●
Quick Oats	82	30g	17	14
ⓖ Quick Steel Cut Oats	53	40g dry	23	12
Vita Brits	68	33g	23	16
Weeties	●	30g	20	●

★ little or no carbs ■ high in saturated fat ● untested/unknown ⓖ GI Symbol partner
Low GI = less than or equal to 55

BREAKFAST CEREALS

FOOD	GI	SAMPLE SERVING	AVAILABLE CARB (g) PER SERVE	GL PER SERVE
Vogel's				
Grain Clusters, classic	54	45g	29	15
Muesli Cluster Spice	51	45g	27	14
Muesli Fruit & Nut	48	45g	24	12
Ultra-Bran	45	45g	22	10
Woolworth's Select				
Natural Swiss Bircher muesli	52	½ cup, 50g	30	16
Naytura Fruit & Nut muesli	48	30g	14	7

Note: For liquid breakfasts/breakfast beverages, see products listed in Beverages: Milkshakes, smoothies & sports drinks

★ little or no carbs ■ high in saturated fat ● untested/unknown ⓒ GI Symbol partner
Low GI = less than or equal to 55

DAIRY PRODUCTS

FOOD	GI	SAMPLE SERVING	AVAILABLE CARB (g) PER SERVE	GL PER SERVE
Milk				
Regular, whole, 4% fat	27–34	1 cup, 250ml	12	4
Dairy Farmers	31	1 cup, 250ml	12	4
Fat-reduced, 1–2% fat	20–30	1 cup, 250ml	15	4
Farmer's Best with Omega-3, Dairy Farmers	27	1 cup, 250ml	19	5
HiLo, Pura Masters	20	1 cup, 250ml	13	3
Lite Start, Pura	30	1 cup, 250ml	13	4
Lite White, Dairy Farmers	30	1 cup, 250ml	14	4
Skim, <1% fat,	20–34	1 cup, 250ml	12	3
Dairy Farmers	32	1 cup, 250ml	12	4
Shape, calcium-enriched	34	1 cup, 250ml	17	6
Skimmer, Pura	20	1 cup, 250ml	12	2
Tone, Pura	30	1 cup, 250ml	14	4
Buttermilk	●	1 cup, 250ml	6	●

★ little or no carbs ■ high in saturated fat ● untested/unknown ☺ GI Symbol partner
Low GI = less than or equal to 55

DAIRY PRODUCTS

FOOD	GI	SAMPLE SERVING	AVAILABLE CARB (g) PER SERVE	GL PER SERVE
Other milk products				
Cheese	★	40g	0	●
Condensed milk, canned, skim	●	½ cup, 125ml	75	●
Condensed milk, canned, whole	61	½ cup, 125ml	69	42
Evaporated milk, canned, whole	●	½ cup, 125ml	13	●
Powdered milk, whole, dry powder	●	4 tbsp, 30g	11	●
Powdered milk, skim, dry powder	●	2 tbsp, heaped, 25g	13	●
Fermented milk drink, Yakult	46	1 bottle, 65ml	12	6
Fermented milk drink, Yakult Light	36	1 bottle, 65ml	9	3
Flavoured milk				
Big M, banana	29	1 carton, 600ml	53	15
Big M, chocolate or strawberry	37	1 cup, 250ml	24–25	9
Big M, iced coffee	29	1 small carton, 300ml	27	8
Feelgood Chocolate	23	1 small carton, 300ml	16	4

★ little or no carbs ■ high in saturated fat ● untested/unknown ⓒ GI Symbol partner
Low GI = less than or equal to 55

DAIRY PRODUCTS

FOOD	GI	SAMPLE SERVING	AVAILABLE CARB (g) PER SERVE	GL PER SERVE
Flavoured milk (continued)				
Feelgood Coffee	27	1 small carton, 300ml	16	4
Full fat, banana, honey & malt flavoured	31	300ml	32	10
Commercial, low fat, artificially sweetened	24	300ml	18	4
Commercial, low fat, sugar sweetened	34	300ml	22	7
☻ Malted milk powder, Nestlé, 20g in full fat milk	45	200ml	24	11
Malt Milo powder, Nestlé, 20g in full fat milk	37	¾ cup, 200ml	24	9
☻ 20g in reduced fat milk	40	200ml	25	10
☻ 20g in skim milk	46	200ml	24	11
Masters varieties				
Iced Coffee Espresso	29	1 small carton, 300ml	24	7
Iced Coffee light milk	29	1 small carton, 300ml	22	6
Iced Coffee One	29	1 carton, 600ml	34	10
Mocha full fat milk	32	1 carton, 600ml	62	20
Mocha One	27	1 carton, 600ml	40	11
Light, 99% fat free, chocolate or mocha flavour	27	1 carton, 600ml	49–55	14
Reduced fat, chocolate or strawberry flavour	35	1 small carton, 300ml	29	10

★ little or no carbs ■ high in saturated fat ● untested/unknown ☻ GI Symbol partner
Low GI = less than or equal to 55

DAIRY PRODUCTS

FOOD	GI	SAMPLE SERVING	AVAILABLE CARB (g) PER SERVE	GL PER SERVE
Flavoured milk (continued)				
Milo powder, Nestlé,				
20g in full fat milk	33	¾ cup, 200ml	24	8
ⓖ 20g in reduced fat milk	36	200ml	24	9
ⓖ 20g in skim milk	39	200ml	24	9
ⓖ Milo Ready-to-drink Tetra pack,				
Nestlé	34	200ml	22	7
Nesquik powder, 12g in reduced fat milk				
Chocolate flavour	41	¾ cup, 200ml	21	9
Strawberry flavour	35	¾ cup, 200ml	22	8
Pauls Good to Go Fruit Smoothie				
Mango Passionfruit	25	1 cup, 250ml	32	8
Mixed Berry	30	1 cup, 250ml	32	10
Strawberry	30	1 cup, 250ml	32	10
Tropical	25	1 cup, 250ml	32	8
Rush, low fat, Heavenly				
Malt Vanilla, Ultimate				
Chocolate, Wicked Latte	26–31	1 bottle, 500ml	27–30	7–9
Smoothie varieties				
banana	30	1 cup, 250ml	26	8
fruit	35	1 cup, 250ml	30	11
mango	32	1 cup, 250ml	27	9
Sustagen varieties				
ⓖ Dutch Chocolate, Vanilla	31	1 carton, 250ml	41	13
ⓖ Sport drink	43	2 scoops in water, 40g	26	11

★ little or no carbs ■ high in saturated fat ● untested/unknown ⓖ GI Symbol partner
Low GI = less than or equal to 55

DAIRY PRODUCTS

FOOD	GI	SAMPLE SERVING	AVAILABLE CARB (g) PER SERVE	GL PER SERVE
Yoghurt				
Generic Yoghurt				
Natural, plain, unflavoured,				
low fat	14	½ cup, 125g	8	1
flavoured	41	1 tub, 200g	24	10
Flavoured, low fat, artificially				
sweetened	20	½ cup, 125g	7	1
Brownes Diet No Fat,				
various flavours	24–40	1 tub, 200g	15	4–6
Dairy Dream				
Diet Deli Natural Yoghurt	17	1 tub, 95g	10	2
Diet Deli Yoghurt				
with Passionfruit	21	1 tub, 95g	10	2
Diet Deli Yoghurt				
with Raspberry	21	1 tub, 95g	9	2
Dairy Farmers Thick and Creamy				
98% Fat Free, various				
flavours	31–32	1 tub, 170g	26	8
Light, various flavours	29–33	1 tub, 170g	10–11	3–4
Jalna varieties				
Bio Dynamic, bush				
honey flavour	26	½ cup, 125g	16	4
Fat Free, natural	19	½ cup, 125g	9	2

★ little or no carbs ■ high in saturated fat ● untested/unknown ☺ GI Symbol partner
Low GI = less than or equal to 55

138

DAIRY PRODUCTS

FOOD	GI	SAMPLE SERVING	AVAILABLE CARB (g) PER SERVE	GL PER SERVE
Yoghurt (continued)				
Jalna varieties (continued)				
Greek style	12	½ cup, 125g	8	1
Leben European style	11	½ cup, 125g	9	1
Premium Blend,				
creamy vanilla	18	1 tub, 200g	30	5
Tamar Valley Greek No Added				
Sugar Yoghurt, various				
flavours	21	1 tub, 115g	8–10	2
Vaalia Kids Probiotic Yoghurt,				
various flavours	23–27	1 tub, 140g	17	4–5
Vaalia Light Probiotic Yoghurt				
French Vanilla	24	1 tub, 150g	11	3
Vaalia, low fat varieties				
Lemon crème	43	1 tub, 150g	27	12
Luscious berries	28	¾ cup, 200g	31	9
Probiotic Yoghurt				
Apple Crumble	33	1 tub, 160g	26	9
Probiotic Yoghurt				
Apricot Mango				
Peach	28	1 tub, 100g	15	4
Probiotic Yoghurt				
French Vanilla	34	1 tub, 100g	17	6

★ little or no carbs ■ high in saturated fat ● untested/unknown © GI Symbol partner
Low GI = less than or equal to 55

DAIRY PRODUCTS

FOOD	GI	SAMPLE SERVING	AVAILABLE CARB (g) PER SERVE	GL PER SERVE
Yoghurt (continued)				
Vaalia, low fat varieties (continued)				
Probiotic Yoghurt				
Vanilla Blueberry	30	1 tub, 100g	16	5
Passionfruit	32	1 tub, 175g	29	9
Strawberry	28	1 tub, 175g	28	8
Yoplait varieties				
Lite, all flavours	25–37	1 tub, 175g	23–29	8
Forme, various flavours	26–33	1 tub, 175g	9–11	2–4
Forme Satisfy, various flavours	24–27	1 tub, 170g	11–14	3–4
Go Gurt, various flavours	39–44	1 tube, 70g	10	4
Petit Miam Apple Pear Cinnamon	41	1 tub, 100g	14	6
Petit Miam Banana	39	1 tub, 100g	14	5
Petit Miam Blueberry	43	1 tub, 100g	14	6
Petit Miam Fruit Salad	41	1 tub, 100g	14	6
Petit Miam Mixed Berry	43	1 tub, 100g	14	6
Petit Miam Strawberry	43	1 tub, 100g	14	6
Petit Miam Strawberry & Banana	39	1 tub, 100g	14	5
Petit Miam Vanilla	38	1 tub, 100g	14	5
Squeezie Pouch, Banana	44	1 pouch, 70g	10	4
Squeezie Pouch, Blueberry	42	1 pouch, 70g	10	4

★ little or no carbs ■ high in saturated fat ● untested/unknown ☺ GI Symbol partner
Low GI = less than or equal to 55

DAIRY PRODUCTS

FOOD	GI	SAMPLE SERVING	AVAILABLE CARB (g) PER SERVE	GL PER SERVE
Custard				
Homemade, from custard powder, with milk and sugar	43	½ cup, 125ml	14	6
Low fat, vanilla flavoured, Nestlé	29	½ cup, 125ml	19	5
Paul's Trim, vanilla, reduced fat	37	½ cup, 125ml	19	7
Yogo Choc Rock Chocolate Custard	43	1 tub, 150g	25	11
Yoplait Petit Miam varieties				
Choc Banana Custard	43	1 tub, 100g	16	7
Choc Berry Custard	43	1 tub, 100g	16	7
Chocolate Custard	43	1 tub, 100g	17	7
Ice-cream				
Paddlepop varieties				
banana, chocolate, rainbow	50–52	1 serve, 68ml	11	6
Moo, chocolate	48	1 serve, 68ml	13	6
Moo, strawberry	51	1 serve, 68ml	14	7
Sara Lee, French vanilla, ultra chocolate flavour	38	2 scoops, 100g	18	7
Vanilla	47	2 scoops, 100g	21	10

★ little or no carbs ■ high in saturated fat ● untested/unknown © GI Symbol partner
Low GI = less than or equal to 55

DAIRY PRODUCTS

FOOD	GI	SAMPLE SERVING	AVAILABLE CARB (g) PER SERVE	GL PER SERVE
Ice-cream, reduced fat				
Chocollo, low fat Wendy's, in waffle cone	55	100g	22	18
☺ Golden North Diet Plus Vanilla	39	2 scoops, 100g	18	7
☺ Golden North Good & Creamy Vanilla	31	49g	9	3
☺ Golden North Good & Creamy Wild Berries	34	49g	9	3
☺ Golden North Good & Creamy Lemoncello	32	49g	9	3
Light, low fat, vanilla, Peter's	46	2 scoops, 100g	30	14
Low carbohydate, chocolate	32	2 scoops, 100g	4	1
Low fat, low sugar, Peter's No Sugar Added	●	2 scoops, 100g	8	●
Vanilla, low fat (1.2% fat), Norco	47	2 scoops, 100g	20	9
Frozen yoghurt				
Vanilla	46	½ cup, 125ml	21	10

★ little or no carbs ■ high in saturated fat ● untested/unknown ☺ GI Symbol partner
Low GI = less than or equal to 55

DAIRY PRODUCTS

FOOD	GI	SAMPLE SERVING	AVAILABLE CARB (g) PER SERVE	GL PER SERVE
Dairy desserts				
Aero Mousse	37	1 tub, 62g	10	4
Fromage frais	35	1 tub, 125g	15	5
Instant pudding, packet mix made with whole milk, chocolate or vanilla	47	100g	16	8
Yoplait Le Rice				
Apple cinnamon	52	1 tub, 150g	28	15
Cappucino	46	1 tub, 150g	28	13
Chocolate	●	1 tub, 150g	27	●
Classic vanilla	43	1 tub, 150g	27	12
Mocha	46	1 tub, 150g	29	13
Raspberry & white chocolate	51	1 tub, 150g	27	14
Smooth caramel	41	1 tub, 150g	29	12
Strawberry	51	1 tub, 150g	28	14
Tropical mango	54	1 tub, 150g	28	15
Fruche				
Strawberry fields	●	1 tub, 150g	23	●
Tropical mango	●	1 tub, 150g	24	●
Vanilla Bean	49	1 tub, 150g	24	12
Vanilla on mixed berries	49	1 tub, 150g	26	13

★ little or no carbs ■ high in saturated fat ● untested/unknown Ⓖ GI Symbol partner
Low GI = less than or equal to 55

DAIRY PRODUCTS

FOOD	GI	SAMPLE SERVING	AVAILABLE CARB (g) PER SERVE	GL PER SERVE
Milk alternatives				
Almond milk	25	1 cup, 250ml	2	1
Oat milk, Vitasoy	69	1 cup, 250ml	23	16
Quinoa milk with chia, Freedom Foods Ancient Grains	42	1 cup, 250ml	11	5
Rice milk				
Australia's Own, low fat	92	1 cup, 250ml	34	31
Vitasoy rice milk, original	79	1 cup, 250ml	24	19
Soy milk, low fat	●	1 cup, 250ml	15	●
Flavoured soy milk				
Sanitarium				
So Good, Regular	37	250ml	13	5
So Good, Essentials	51	250ml	16	8
Up & Go, soy & cereal liquid breakfast	43–46	1 cup, 250ml	24–26	11
Up & Go Vive Banana	34	1 cup, 250ml	23	8
Up & Go Vive Wild Berry	42	1 cup, 250ml	27	11

★ little or no carbs ■ high in saturated fat ● untested/unknown ⓖ GI Symbol partner
Low GI = less than or equal to 55

DAIRY PRODUCTS

FOOD	GI	SAMPLE SERVING	AVAILABLE CARB (g) PER SERVE	GL PER SERVE
Flavoured soy milk (continued)				
Vita Go				
Banana Honey	29	1 cup, 250ml	29	8
Chocolate	29	1 cup, 250ml	29	8
Vanilla	29	1 cup, 250ml	28	8
Vitasoy reduced fat				
chocolate or vanilla	31	1 cup, 250ml	17–19	5–6
Vitasoy Soy Milky				
Chocolate	31	1 cup, 250ml	19	2
Soy milk				
Fresh-Vitasoy, Calci Plus	24	1 cup, 250ml	15	4
Fresh-Vitasoy, High Fibre	27	1 cup, 250ml	14	4
Vitasoy Light	34	1 cup, 250ml	7	2
Vitasoy, Soy Milky Lite	17	1 cup, 250ml	8	1
Vitasoy, Soy Milky Regular	21	1 cup, 250ml	8	2
Vitasoy, Vitality for				
Women (UHT)	18	1 cup, 250ml	9	2

★ little or no carbs ■ high in saturated fat ● untested/unknown ⓒ GI Symbol partner
Low GI = less than or equal to 55

FRUIT

FOOD	GI	SAMPLE SERVING	AVAILABLE CARB (g) PER SERVE	GL PER SERVE
Fresh				
© Apple, unpeeled	38	1 medium, 166g	18	7
Apricot, raw	34	2 regular, 112g	8	3
Avocado	★	120g	0	0
Banana	52	1 medium, 120g	24	12
© Banana, Ladyfinger	49–53	1 medium, 140g	26	13
Blackberries	●	10 regular, 50g	4	●
Blueberries	53	½ cup, 80g	9	5
Breadfruit	62	¼ cup, 55g	15	9
Cherries	63	1 cup, 124g	15	9
Custard apple	54	1 regular, 320g	52	28
Fig, raw, fresh, unpeeled	●	1 large, 64g	5	●
Fruit salad, fresh, with melon	●	1 cup, 200g	19	●
Grapefruit	25	1 medium, 200g	7	2
© Grapes	53	⅔ cups, 112g	17	9
Guava	●	1 regular, 90g	3	●

★ little or no carbs ■ high in saturated fat ● untested/unknown © GI Symbol partner
Low GI = less than or equal to 55

FRUIT

FOOD	GI	SAMPLE SERVING	AVAILABLE CARB (g) PER SERVE	GL PER SERVE
Fresh (continued)				
Honeydew melon	●	1 cup, 180g	12	●
Kiwifruit	53	1 regular, 95g	9	5
Lemon	★	1 cup, 40g	0	●
Lime	★	1 cup, 40g	0	●
Loquat	●	5 large, 100g	5	●
Lychees, B3 variety	57	7 regular, 90g	15	9
Mandarin	●	1 medium, 86g	7	●
Mango	51	1 regular, 200g	26	13
Mulberries	●	1 cup, 148g	6	●
Nashi pear	●	1 medium, 190g	21	●
Nectarine	43	1 small, 90g	7	3
Orange	42	1 large, 190g	15	16
Paw paw	56	1 cup cubed, 148g	10	6
Peach	42	1 medium, 145g	9	4
☺ Pear, unpeeled	38	1 medium, 166g	22	8
Pear, Williams Bartlett, unpeeled	33	120g	11	4

★ little or no carbs ■ high in saturated fat ● untested/unknown ☺ GI Symbol partner
Low GI = less than or equal to 55

FRUIT

FOOD	GI	SAMPLE SERVING	AVAILABLE CARB (g) PER SERVE	GL PER SERVE
Fresh (continued)				
Persimmon	●	1 medium, 168g	27	●
Pineapple	59	1 cup, diced, 164g	13	8
Plum	39	2 regular, 130g	10	4
Pomegranate, peeled	●	100g	14	●
Prickly pear, peeled	●	100g	9	●
Quince, peeled	●	1 medium, 390g	43	●
Rambutan	●	100g	16	●
Rockmelon/cantaloupe	68	1 cup diced, 190g	8	7
Raspberries	●	100g	7	●
Rhubarb	★	125g	0	●
Strawberries	40	1 punnet, 250g	8	3
Tamarillo, peeled	●	100g	3	●
Tangelo, peeled	●	100g	8	●
Watermelon	78	100g	3	2

★ little or no carbs ■ high in saturated fat ● untested/unknown ⓖ GI Symbol partner
Low GI = less than or equal to 55

FRUIT

FOOD	GI	SAMPLE SERVING	AVAILABLE CARB (g) PER SERVE	GL PER SERVE
Dried				
Apple	29	4 rings, 25g	16	5
Apricot	31	10 halves, 35g	16	5
ⓒ Apricot, Turkish dried, Coles	31	10 halves, 35g	16	5
Cranberries, sweetened	62	2 tbsp, 25g	16	10
Currants	●	2 tbsp, 24g	16	●
Dates	39–45	5 regular, 25g	17	7
Fig	61	2 regular, 20g	21	13
Fruit & nut mix	15	¼ cup, 50g	24	4
Mixed fruit	●	100g	65	●
Peach	35	3 halves, 40g	16	6
Pear	43	1 half, 18g	11	5
Prunes	40	4 regular, 32g	14	6
Raisins	56	1½ tbsp, 20g	16	9
Sultanas	56	1½ tbsp, 20g	15	8

★ little or no carbs   ■ high in saturated fat   ● untested/unknown   ⓒ GI Symbol partner
Low GI = less than or equal to 55

FRUIT

FOOD	GI	SAMPLE SERVING	AVAILABLE CARB (g) PER SERVE	GL PER SERVE
Dried (continued)				
Sunmuscats, Sunbeam	53	¼ cup, 50g	32	17
Tropical fruit & nut mix	49	¼ cup, 50g	14	7
Canned				
Apple, canned, Woolworth's Select	42	½ cup, 125g	10	4
Apricot, canned in light syrup	64	4 halves, 90g	12	8
Apricot, canned in natural juice	51	4 halves, 72g	8	4
Cherries, sour, pitted	41	¼ cup, 130g	12	5
Fruit salad, canned in juice	54	1 cup, 260g	26	14
Grapefruit, ruby red segments canned in juice, Woolworth's Select	47	½ cup, 120g	21	10
Lychees, canned in syrup, drained	79	7 regular, 90g	16	13
Mandarin, segments, canned in fruit juice	47	½ cup,130g	18	8

★ little or no carbs   ■ high in saturated fat   ● untested/unknown   ☺ GI Symbol partner
Low GI = less than or equal to 55

FRUIT

FOOD	GI	SAMPLE SERVING	AVAILABLE CARB (g) PER SERVE	GL PER SERVE
Canned (continued)				
Orange & grapefruit segments, canned in fruit juice, Woolworth's Select	53	½ cup, 120g	19	10
⒢ Coles Australian Apricot Halves 410g (53% Apricots)	44	½ cup, 125g	19	8
⒢ Coles Australian Peach Slices 410g	45	½ cup, 125g	18	8
⒢ Coles Australian Pear Halves 825g	37	½ cup, 125g	17	6
⒢ Coles Australian Pear Slices 410g	37	½ cup, 125g	17	6
⒢ Coles Australian Two Fruits 410g	40	½ cup, 125g	18	7
⒢ Coles Australian Whole Plums 825g	39	½ cup, 125g	19	7
⒢ Coles Fruit Salad 410g	51	½ cup, 125g	16	8
Peach, canned in light syrup	57	½ cup, 132g	17	10
Peach, canned in natural juice	45	½ cup, 132g	12	5

★ little or no carbs ■ high in saturated fat ● untested/unknown ⒢ GI Symbol partner
Low GI = less than or equal to 55

FRUIT

FOOD	GI	SAMPLE SERVING	AVAILABLE CARB (g) PER SERVE	GL PER SERVE
Canned (continued)				
Peaches & grapes, canned in fruit juice, Woolworth's Select	46	½ cup, 120g	12	6
Peaches & pineapple, canned in fruit juice, Woolworth's Select	45	½ cup, 120g	13	6
Pear, canned in fruit juice	43	½ cup, 120g	13	6
Pear, halves, canned in reduced sugar syrup, SPC Lite	25	½ cup, 120g	14	4
Pineapple, canned in juice, drained, Woolworth's Select	43	1 cup, 200g	20	9
Pineapple pieces, canned in fruit juice	49	½ cup, 128g	13	6
Pineapple & papaya pieces, canned in fruit juice, Woolworth's Select	53	½ cup, 120g	17	9

★ little or no carbs ■ high in saturated fat ● untested/unknown ☺ GI Symbol partner
Low GI = less than or equal to 55

LEGUMES

FOOD	GI	SAMPLE SERVING	AVAILABLE CARB (g) PER SERVE	GL PER SERVE
Baked beans				
Canned in tomato sauce	52	½ cup, 150g	18	9
Heinz varieties, canned				
Barbecue sauce	47	1 sml can, 220g	34	16
Cheesy tomato sauce	44	1 sml can, 220g	28	12
Ham sauce	53	1 sml can, 220g	31	16
Mild curry sauce	49	1 sml can, 220g	34	17
Sweet chilli sauce	46	1 sml can, 220g	33	15
Tomato sauce	49	1 sml can, 220g	30	15
Black-eyed beans				
soaked, boiled	42	½ cup, 75g	17	7
Borlotti beans				
Canned, drained, Edgell	41	½ cup, 75g	12	5
Butter beans				
Soaked, boiled	26	½ cup, 75g	8	2
Canned, drained, Edgell	36	½ cup, 80g	11	4
Cannellini beans				
Canned, drained, Edgell	31	½ cup, 128g	15	5

★ little or no carbs ■ high in saturated fat ● untested/unknown © GI Symbol partner
Low GI = less than or equal to 55

LEGUMES

FOOD	GI	SAMPLE SERVING	AVAILABLE CARB (g) PER SERVE	GL PER SERVE
Chickpeas				
Canned, drained	40	½ cup, 80g	11	4
Canned, drained, Edgell	38	1 can, 75g	13	5
Hommus, Chris' Traditional	22	2 tbsp, 40g	3	1
Four-bean mix				
Canned, drained, Edgell	37	1 can, 75g	12	4
Lentils				
Boiled	33	½ cup, 88g	12	4
Brown, canned	42	½ cup, 80g	13	5
© Coles Simply green lentils, dried, boiled	30	⅔ cup, 125g	17	5
Green, dried, boiled	30	⅔ cup, 125g	17	5
Green, canned	48	⅔ cup, 135g	17	8
Red, dried, boiled	26	⅔ cup, 125g	18	5
Red, dried, split, boiled 25 min	21	125g	15	3
Dhal	●	1 cup, 195g	29	●
Mung beans				
Boiled	39	⅔ cup, 125g	15	4

★ little or no carbs ■ high in saturated fat ● untested/unknown © GI Symbol partner
Low GI = less than or equal to 55

LEGUMES

FOOD	GI	SAMPLE SERVING	AVAILABLE CARB (g) PER SERVE	GL PER SERVE
Red kidney beans				
Dried, boiled	51	100g	9	5
Canned, drained, Edgell	36	1 can, 75g	11	4
Pinto beans				
Refried, canned, Casa Fiesta	38	½ cup, 115g	20	8
Steamed	33	½ cup, 150g	23	8
Snake beans				
Snake beans	★	70g	0	●
Soy beans				
Dried, boiled	18	1 cup, 170g	4	1
Canned, drained, Edgell	14	½ cup, 100g	3	0
Split peas				
Dried, boiled, yellow/green	25	1 cup, 180g	13	3

★ little or no carbs   ■ high in saturated fat   ● untested/unknown   ⓖ GI Symbol partner
Low GI = less than or equal to 55

MEAT, SEAFOOD & PROTEIN

FOOD	GI	SAMPLE SERVING	AVAILABLE CARB (g) PER SERVE	GL PER SERVE
Bacon	★■	50g	0	●
Beef, lean	★	120g	0	●
Brawn	★■	75g	0	●
Calamari rings, squid, not battered or crumbed	★	70g	0	●
Chicken, no skin	★	110g	0	●
Duck	★■	140g	0	●
Eggs	★■	120g	0	●
Fish	★	120g	0	●
Ham, lean	★	24g	0	●
Lamb	★	120g	0	●
Liver Sausage	★■	30g	0	●
Liverwurst	★■	30g	0	●
Oysters, natural, plain	★	85g	0	●
Pork, lean	★	120g	0	●
Prawns	★	150g	0	●
Salami	★■	120g	0	●

★ little or no carbs   ■ high in saturated fat   ● untested/unknown   ☻ GI Symbol partner
Low GI = less than or equal to 55

MEAT, SEAFOOD & PROTEIN

FOOD	GI	SAMPLE SERVING	AVAILABLE CARB (g) PER SERVE	GL PER SERVE
Salmon, fresh or canned in water or brine	★	150g	0	●
Sardines	★	60g	0	●
Sausages, fried	28■	100g	3	1
Scallops, natural, plain	★	160g	0	●
Shellfish	★	120g	0	●
Steak, lean	★	120g	0	●
Tofu, bean curd, plain, unsweetened	★	100g	0	●
Trout, fresh or frozen	★	63g	0	●
Tuna, fresh or canned in water or brine	★	120g	0	●
Turkey, lean	★	140g	0	●
Veal	★	120g	0	●

★ little or no carbs ■ high in saturated fat ● untested/unknown © GI Symbol partner
Low GI = less than or equal to 55

RICE, PASTA, NOODLES & GRAINS

FOOD	GI	SAMPLE SERVING	AVAILABLE CARB (g) PER SERVE	GL PER SERVE
Barley				
Pearl, boiled	25	1 cup, 190g	40	10
Bulgur (burghul or cracked wheat)				
Ⓖ Coles Fine Grit Bourghal	47	100g	28	13
Soaked in water	48	100g	28	13
Buckwheat				
Groats, boiled	54	1 cup, 180g	34	18
Cornmeal/polenta				
Boiled	68	1 cup, 250g	22	15
Couscous				
Cooked, soaked	65	1 cup, 160g	15	10
Ⓖ Blu Gourmet pearl couscous, cooked	52	½ cup	19	10
Ⓖ Blu Gourmet pearl couscous, wholemeal	53	⅓ cup	31	16
Flours				
Wheat, white	●	1 tbsp, 13g	8	●
Wheat, wholemeal	●	1 tbsp, 13g	8	●

★ little or no carbs ■ high in saturated fat ● untested/unknown Ⓖ GI Symbol partner
Low GI = less than or equal to 55

RICE, PASTA, NOODLES & GRAINS

FOOD	GI	SAMPLE SERVING	AVAILABLE CARB (g) PER SERVE	GL PER SERVE
Flours (continued)				
Millet, boiled	71	100g	23	16
Noodles				
Asian, shelf stable noodles e.g. Hokkien, Singapore	●	½ pkt, 110g	35	●
Buckwheat noodles	59	180g	42	25
Herman Brot low carb high protein noodles	22	80g dry	13	3
Instant 2-Minute Noodles, Maggi, 99% fat free	67	1 pkt, 380g	56	38
Mung bean noodles, Lungkow bean thread, dried, boiled	39	1 cup, 180g	45	18
Rice noodles, fresh, boiled	40	1 cup, 180g	39	16
Rice pasta, brown, boiled	92	1 cup, 180g	38	35
Rice vermicelli, dried, boiled	58	¼ pkt, 250g	50	29
Soba noodles, instant, served in soup	46	1 cup, 180g	49	23
Udon, plain	62	½ pkt, 200g	50	31

★ little or no carbs ■ high in saturated fat ● untested/unknown ⓒ GI Symbol partner
Low GI = less than or equal to 55

RICE, PASTA, NOODLES & GRAINS

FOOD	GI	SAMPLE SERVING	AVAILABLE CARB (g) PER SERVE	GL PER SERVE
Quinoa				
Coles				
Ⓖ Simply Gluten Free Mexican Style Quinoa and Brown Rice Cups	49	1 pouch, 125g	43	21
Ⓖ Simply Gluten Free Quinoa Cups	53	1 pouch, 125g	50	27
Ⓖ Simply Organic Quinoa Grain Black	53	⅓ cup, 62g	13	7
Ⓖ Simply Organic Quinoa Grain Red	53	⅓ cup, 62g	13	7
Ⓖ Simply Organic Quinoa Grain Tricolour	53	⅓ cup, 62g	13	7
Ⓖ Simply Organic Quinoa Grain White	53	⅓ cup, 62g	13	7
Boiled, Nature First Organic	53	⅓ cup, 62g	13	7
Rice				
Arborio/risotto rice, boiled, SunRice	69	1 cup, 170g	49	34
Basmati rice, white, boiled	58	1 cup, 170g	47	27

★ little or no carbs ■ high in saturated fat ● untested/unknown Ⓖ GI Symbol partner
Low GI = less than or equal to 55

RICE, PASTA, NOODLES & GRAINS

FOOD	GI	SAMPLE SERVING	AVAILABLE CARB (g) PER SERVE	GL PER SERVE
Rice (continued)				
Basmati rice, white, SunRice, boiled	59	I cup, 170g	44	26
☺ Basmati rice, white, SunRice, microwave pouch	52	125g	35	18
Broken rice, Thai, white, cooked in rice cooker	86	I cup, 170g	49	42
Brown rice, boiled/Pelde (Sungold)	86	I cup, 170g	43	37
Calrose rice, brown, medium-grain, boiled	76	I cup, 170g	45	34
Calrose rice, white, medium-grain, boiled	87	I cup, 170g	48	42
☺ Coles Brown Rice and Chia Seeds	41	125g	53	22
☺ Coles Brown Rice and Quinoa	51	125g	56	29
☺ Coles 7 Ancient Grains	49	125g	56	28
☺ Coles Mexican Style Rice	47	125g	42	20
Glutinous rice, white, cooked in rice cooker	98	½ cup, 170g	36	35

★ little or no carbs ■ high in saturated fat ● untested/unknown ☺ GI Symbol partner
Low GI = less than or equal to 55

RICE, PASTA, NOODLES & GRAINS

FOOD	GI	SAMPLE SERVING	AVAILABLE CARB (g) PER SERVE	GL PER SERVE
Rice (continued)				
Instant rice, white, cooked 6 min with water	87	1 cup, 170g	48	42
Japanese-style sushi rice, SunRice	73	1 cup, 170g	46	34
Jasmine fragrant rice, SunRice	89	1 cup, 170g	45	40
Koshihikari rice, white, SunRice, boiled	61	1 cup, 170g	43	26
Long-grain rice, white, boiled 15 min, Mahatma	50	1 cup, 170g	46	23
☺ SunRice low GI brown rice	51	1 cup, 170g	50	25
Medium-grain, brown, SunRice	59	1 cup, 170g	49	29
Parboiled rice, Pelde, Sungold	87	1 cup, 170g	49	43
Sri Lankan Red Rice, boiled	59	1 cup, 170g	45	27
Sunbrown Quick rice, Ricegrowers, boiled	80	1 cup, 170g	43	34
☺ SunRice Doongara low GI Clever rice	53	1 cup, 170g	53	28
Uncle Ben's Express Long Grain Rice	59	125g	39	23
Uncle Ben's Express Microwave Basmati Rice	63	100g	30	19

★ little or no carbs ■ high in saturated fat ● untested/unknown ☺ GI Symbol partner
Low GI = less than or equal to 55

RICE, PASTA, NOODLES & GRAINS

FOOD	GI	SAMPLE SERVING	AVAILABLE CARB (g) PER SERVE	GL PER SERVE
Rice (continued)				
Uncle Ben's Microwave Long Grain Rice	59	100g	31	18
White long-grain rice, Premium, SunRice	59	1 cup, 170g	45	27
Wild rice, boiled	57	½ cup, 75g	15	9
Pasta				
Capellini	45	1 cup, 150g	45	20
Fettucine, egg	40	1 cup, 180g	46	18
Fusilli twists, tricolour	51	1 cup, 150g	42	21
Gnocchi, cooked	68	100g	29	20
Lasagne, beef, commercial	47	200g	30	14
Latina Fresh Pasta				
Agnolotti, ricotta & spinach	47	½ pkt, 280g	83	39
Fettucine, egg	54	½ pkt, 360g	92	50
Lasagne sheets	49	1 regular, 47g	23	11
Ravioli, beef	43	½ pkt, 315g	70	30
Ravioli, chicken & garlic	44	½ pkt, 279g	76	33
Ravioli, wholegrain, ricotta & spinach	39	½ pkt, 220g	58	23
Tortellini, mixed veal	48	½ pkt, 305g	80	38

★ little or no carbs ■ high in saturated fat ● untested/unknown ⓒ GI Symbol partner
Low GI = less than or equal to 55

RICE, PASTA, NOODLES & GRAINS

FOOD	GI	SAMPLE SERVING	AVAILABLE CARB (g) PER SERVE	GL PER SERVE
Pasta (continued)				
Vetta varieties				
High fibre range	45	100g	66	30
Lasagne sheets	53	I regular, 19g	13	7
Macaroni, boiled 8–10 min	49	I cup, 150g	40	20
Spaghetti, boiled 8–10 min	49	I cup, 180g	48	24
Macaroni	47	I cup, 150g	40	19
Macaroni & Cheese, prepared, Kraft	64	approx. I cup, 70g	47	30
Spaghetti	44	I cup, 180g	48	21
Spaghetti, protein-enriched	27	I cup, 180g	14	
Spaghetti, wholemeal	42	I cup, 180g	42	18
Spirali, white, durum wheat	43	I cup, 150g	44	19
Star Pastina, white, boiled 5 min	38	I cup, 150g	48	18
Vermicelli	35	I cup, 180g	48	17
Instant pasta				
Pasta & Sauce, prepared, Woolworth's Select	48–57	¼ pkt, 110g	20–23	10–12

★ little or no carbs ■ high in saturated fat ● untested/unknown ☺ GI Symbol partner
Low GI = less than or equal to 55

RICE, PASTA, NOODLES & GRAINS

FOOD	GI	SAMPLE SERVING	AVAILABLE CARB (g) PER SERVE	GL PER SERVE
Pasta (continued)				
Gluten-free pasta				
Coles Simply Gluten Free varieties				
ⓖ Penne	46	100g (dry)	82	38
ⓖ Spaghetti	46	100g (dry)	83	38
ⓖ Spirals	46	100g (dry)	81	37
Rice pasta, Freedom Foods	51	1 cup, 180g	47	24
Corn pasta, Orgran	78	1 cup, 180g	42	33
Rice and maize pasta, Ris'O'Mais, Orgran	76	1 cup, 180g	49	37
Spaghetti, canned in tomato sauce, Orgran	68	1 can, 220g	27	18
Semolina				
Cooked	55	1 cup, 245g	17	10
Spelt				
Dry	●	100g	59	●
Cooked	●	100g	23	●

★ little or no carbs ■ high in saturated fat ● untested/unknown ⓖ GI Symbol partner
Low GI = less than or equal to 55

RICE, PASTA, NOODLES & GRAINS

FOOD	GI	SAMPLE SERVING	AVAILABLE CARB (g) PER SERVE	GL PER SERVE
Wheat				
Wheat bran, unprocessed	●	100g	16	●
Wheatgerm	●	100g	30	●
Whole wheat kernels, cooked	52	50g (dry)	37	19
Rye				
Whole rye kernels, cooked	39	50g (dry)	38	15

★ little or no carbs ■ high in saturated fat ● untested/unknown ⊚ GI Symbol partner
Low GI = less than or equal to 55

SNACKFOODS & TREATS

FOOD	GI	SAMPLE SERVING	AVAILABLE CARB (g) PER SERVE	GL PER SERVE
Cakes & pastries				
Angel food cake	67	1 sml piece, 57g	31	21
Banana cake, homemade	51	1 slice, 80g	38	19
Bavarian, chocolate honeycomb lite, Sara Lee	31	¼ cake, 93g	25	8
Carrot cake	38	1 sml slice, 50g	19	7
Chinese Moon Cakes	56	1 cake, 80g	50	28
Chinese Pineapple Bun	65	1 bun, 62g	34	22
Chocolate brownies	42■	1 serve, 56g	30	13
Chocolate cake, pkt mix, with frosting, Betty Crocker	38■	1 slice, 110g	52	20
Chocolate mud cake	43■	1 slice, 100g	54	23
Chocolate crackles	43■	1 serve, 12g	12	5
Crumble, apple berry, commercially made	41	1 slice, 165g	34	14
Cupcake, strawberry iced	73■	1 serve, 38g	26	19
Danish, apple & peach, Sara Lee Lite	50	⅙ pkt, 67g	29	15

★ little or no carbs ■ high in saturated fat ● untested/unknown © GI Symbol partner
Low GI = less than or equal to 55

SNACKFOODS & TREATS

FOOD	GI	SAMPLE SERVING	AVAILABLE CARB (g) PER SERVE	GL PER SERVE
Cakes & pastries (continued)				
Egg Tart, Chinese style	45	1 serve, 60g	21	9
Fruit cake, commercial, Big Sister	53■	1 slice, 50g	28	15
Fruit mince pies, Mr Kipling	58■	1 serve, 59g	35	20
Glutinous rice ball	61	1 serve, 220g	95	58
Lamington	87■	1 serve, 50g	29	25
Pavlova, prepared with fresh cream, strawberries, banana and passionfruit	49■	1 slice, 120g	33	16
Pound cake	54■	1 sml slice, 50g	23	12
Puff pastry	56■	100g	40	22
Red Bean dessert	75	1 serve, 200g	38	29
Sponge cake, plain, unfilled	46	1 slice, 25g	14	6
Vanilla cake, from pkt mix with frosting, Betty Crocker	42■	1 slice, 65g	31	13

★ little or no carbs ■ high in saturated fat ● untested/unknown ⓒ GI Symbol partner
Low GI = less than or equal to 55

SNACKFOODS & TREATS

FOOD	GI	SAMPLE SERVING	AVAILABLE CARB (g) PER SERVE	GL PER SERVE
Confectionery				
Chocolate	42–49■	4 sml squares, 24g	15	7
Chocolate-coated almonds	21■	5–6 almonds, 30g	8	2
Chocolate, dark, Dove	23■	4 sml squares, 24g	13	3
Chocolate, fructose sweetened	20■	4 sml squares, 24g	15	3
Chocolate, white, Lindt Lindor	34■	6 pieces, 33g	14	5
Chocolate, white, Milky Bar, Nestlé	44■	1 fun size, 15g	8	4
Gummi confectionery	94	6 pieces, 24g	15	14
Jelly beans	78	10–15 lollies, 30g	28	22
Jelly, diet, made from crystals with water	★	½ cup, 120g	0	●
Jelly, made from commercial jelly crystals	53	½ cup, 120g	19	10
Licorice, soft	78	1 stick, 12g	9	7
Life Savers, peppermint candy, Nestlé	70	1 pkt, 22g	21	15

★ little or no carbs   ■ high in saturated fat   ● untested/unknown   ☺ GI Symbol partner
Low GI = less than or equal to 55

169

SNACKFOODS & TREATS

FOOD	GI	SAMPLE SERVING	AVAILABLE CARB (g) PER SERVE	GL PER SERVE
Confectionery (continued)				
M&M's, peanut, Mars	33■	1 fun size, 14g	8	3
Mars Bar, Mars	62■	1 fun size, 22g	16	10
Marshmallows, plain, pink & white	62	4 small, 20g	16	10
Milkybar Buttons, Nestlé	41■	15 buttons, 20g	11	5
Milky Way bar, Mars	62■	1 fun size, 14g	10	6
Milo bar, Nestlé	40■	1 serve, 21g	15	6
Skittles, fruit candies, Mars	70	1 fun size, 25g	23	16
Rum balls, Woolworth's	50■	1 serve, 25g	14	7
Snickers bar, Mars	41■	1 fun size, 22g	13	5
Twix bar, Mars	44■	1 fun size, 16g	10	4
Yummiees jelly lollies, Allseps	43	4 lollies, 15g	5	2
Muffins				
Apple, homemade	46	1 regular, 60g	29	13
Apple blueberry, Sara Lee	49■	1 regular, 60g	25	12
Apple, oat & sultana	54	1 regular, 50g	26	14

★ little or no carbs   ■ high in saturated fat   ● untested/unknown   ⊙ GI Symbol partner
Low GI = less than or equal to 55

SNACKFOODS & TREATS

FOOD	GI	SAMPLE SERVING	AVAILABLE CARB (g) PER SERVE	GL PER SERVE
Muffins (continued)				
Apricot, coconut & honey	60■	1 regular, 50g	26	16
Banana, oat & honey	65	1 regular, 50g	26	17
Berry, Nut & Seeds lower carb, Muffin Break	29	1 regular, 112g	20	6
Blueberry	59	1 regular, 57g	29	17
Blueberry, Sara Lee	50■	1 regular, 60g	31	16
Bran	60	1 regular, 57g	24	14
Carrot	62	1 regular, 57g	32	20
Chocolate	53■	1 regular, 60g	30	16
Choc-butterscotch	53■	1 regular, 50g	28	15
Choc-chip, Sara Lee	52■	1 regular, 60g	32	17
Double chocolate	46■	1 regular, 60g	34	16
Macadamia, Mango & Passionfruit lower carb, Muffin Break	34	1 regular, 111g	21	7
Oatmeal, from packet mix	69	1 regular, 50g	35	24

★ little or no carbs ■ high in saturated fat ● untested/unknown © GI Symbol partner
Low GI = less than or equal to 55

SNACKFOODS & TREATS

FOOD	GI	SAMPLE SERVING	AVAILABLE CARB (g) PER SERVE	GL PER SERVE
Nuts				
Almonds	●	½ cup, 75g	3	●
Beer nuts	23	½ cup, 100g	22	5
Cashews, natural	22	½ cup, 100g	26	6
Chestnut, roasted	●	5 kernels, 100g	34	●
Dried fruit & nut mix, commercial	32	¼ cup, 50g	22	7
Macadamia	●	½ cup, 75g	3	●
Mixed nuts, roasted, salted	24	½ cup, 100g	25	6
Peanuts, dry roasted	23	½ cup, 100g	22	5
Pecan	10	½ cup, 100g	5	1
Pine nut	●	½ cup, 100g	5	●
Sesame seeds	★	12g	0	●
Walnut	●	½ cup, 53g	<0.5	●
Coles				
☺ Beer nuts	23	½ cup, 100g	22	5
☺ Cashews, dry roasted	22	½ cup, 100g	26	6
☺ Cashews, natural	22	½ cup, 100g	26	6
☺ Cashews, roasted & salted	22	½ cup, 100g	26	6
☺ Mixed nuts	24	½ cup, 100g	25	6

★ little or no carbs ■ high in saturated fat ● untested/unknown ☺ GI Symbol partner
Low GI = less than or equal to 55

172

SNACKFOODS & TREATS

FOOD	GI	SAMPLE SERVING	AVAILABLE CARB (g) PER SERVE	GL PER SERVE
Nuts (continued				
© Mixed nuts, salted	24	½ cup, 100g	25	6
© Peanuts, salted	23	½ cup, 100g	22	5
© Peanuts, unsalted	23	½ cup, 100g	22	5
© Pecans, Australian natural	10	½ cup, 100g	5	1
Savoury snacks				
Burger Rings	90■	1 pkt, 50g	29	26
Chickpea chips, Freedom Foods	44	⅕ pkt, 50g	25	11
Chips, potato	57■	1 mini pkt, 25g	12	7
Corn chips	42■	1 pkt, 50g	26	11
Grain Waves Wholegrain chips, original, Smith's	51	1 pkt, 40g	25	13
Poppin Microwave Popcorn varieties, Green's Foods				
Butter	51	¼ bag, 25g	14	7
Lite	67	1 pkt, 85g	48	32
plain	72	1 cup, 9g	5	4
Prawn cracker	●	1 pkt, 50g	33	●
Pretzels	●	1 cup, 42g	27	●
Pretzels, oven-baked, traditional wheat flavour, Parkers	84	10 pretzels, 19g	15	13

★ little or no carbs ■ high in saturated fat ● untested/unknown © GI Symbol partner
Low GI = less than or equal to 55

SNACKFOODS & TREATS

FOOD	GI	SAMPLE SERVING	AVAILABLE CARB (g) PER SERVE	GL PER SERVE
Savoury snacks (continued)				
Pringles Original potato crisps	57■	16 crisps, 28g	15	9
Rice crackers	91	11 crackers, 19g	15	14
Twisties, Smith's	74■	1 pkt, 30g	19	14
Snack bars				
Bakers Delight, Fit2Go Bars				
Cranberry & Nuts bar	51	1 bar, 77g	25	13
Fruit & Cinnamon bar	53	1 bar, 77g	28	15
Be Natural Four Bars				
Coconut, Apricot,				
Oats & Chia	41	1 bar, 32g	14	6
Currant, Berry, Oats				
& Pepita	48	1 bar, 32g	15	7
Be Natural Nut Bars				
Almond Apricot	44	1 bar, 40g	18	8
Fruit and Nut	38	1 bar, 50g	18	7
Nut Delight	29	1 bar, 40g	11	3
Be Natural Trail Bars				
Dark Chocolate & Nut	55	1 bar, 32g	19	11
Honey Nut	54	1 bar, 32g	19	10

★ little or no carbs ■ high in saturated fat ● untested/unknown Ⓖ GI Symbol partner
Low GI = less than or equal to 55

SNACKFOODS & TREATS

FOOD	GI	SAMPLE SERVING	AVAILABLE CARB (g) PER SERVE	GL PER SERVE
Snack bars (continued)				
Carman's				
Apricot & Almond Muesli Bar	51	1 bar, 45g	23	12
Apricot Muesli Bites	54	1 bar, 20g	12	6
Classic Fruit Muesli Bar	56	1 bar, 45g	25	14
Classic Fruit Muesli Bites	52	20g	12	6
Dark Chocolate, Blueberry Superfoods Bar	52	1 bar, 35g	23	12
Dark Chocolate, Cranberry & Almond Bar	53	1 bar, 35g	19	10
Fruit Bites	52	1 bar, 20g	11	6
Original Fruit-Free Muesli Bar	56	1 bar, 45g	25	14
Super Berry Cranberry, Blueberry & Goji Muesli Bar	50	1 bar, 45g	23	12
Yoghurt, Apricot & Almond Bar	44	1 bar, 35g	18	8
Freedom Foods				
Hi-Lite breakfast bar	53	1 bar, 35g	21	11
Omega Bar, gluten-free, seed & nut	21	1 bar, 40g	17	4
Superberry breakfast bar	54	1 bar, 35g	20	11
Healtheries Simple Snack Bar				
Apricot & yoghurt	40	1 bar, 45g	23	9
Berry & yoghurt	51	1 bar, 45g	24	12
Chocolate	35	1 bar, 45g	25	9
Ironman PR bar, chocolate	39	1 bar, 65g	26	10

★ little or no carbs ■ high in saturated fat ● untested/unknown © GI Symbol partner
Low GI = less than or equal to 55

SNACKFOODS & TREATS

FOOD	GI	SAMPLE SERVING	AVAILABLE CARB (g) PER SERVE	GL PER SERVE
Snack bars (continued)				
Kellogg's Crunchy Nut Nutty				
Mixed Nut Bar	36	1 bar, 30g	14	5
Peanut Bar	34	1 bar, 30g	14	5
Kellogg's K-Time Twists varieties				
Apple & Cinnamon	51	1 bar, 37g	24	12
Raspberry & Apple	55	1 bar, 37g	24	13
Strawberry & Blueberry	45	1 bar, 37g	24	11
Strawberry & Yoghurt	47	1 bar, 37g	24	11
Mother Earth Baked Fruit				
Stick, apricot-filled	50	1 bar, 19g	13	7
ProteinFX LO GI				
Banana Boom bar	48	1 bar, 30g	17	8
Superfruit Slam bar	52	1 bar, 30g	18	9
Roll-Ups, processed fruit				
snack, Uncle Tobys	99	1 serve, 15g	11	11
Trim Low-GI protein snack bar, Aussie Bodies				
Berryliscious	46	1 bar, 50g	15	7
Chocorama	31	1 bar, 50g	14	4

★ little or no carbs　■ high in saturated fat　● untested/unknown　ⓖ GI Symbol partner
Low GI = less than or equal to 55

FOOD	GI	SAMPLE SERVING	AVAILABLE CARB (g) PER SERVE	GL PER SERVE
Snack bars (continued)				
Uncle Tobys Farmer's Pick muesli bar;				
ⓒ Almond & Blueberry	51	1 bar, 31g	17	9
ⓒ Roasted Macadamia & Almond	47	1 bar, 31g	17	8
ⓒ Fig & Apricot	53	1 bar, 31g	18	10

★ little or no carbs ■ high in saturated fat ● untested/unknown ⓒ GI Symbol partner
Low GI = less than or equal to 55

SPREADS & SWEETENERS

FOOD	GI	SAMPLE SERVING	AVAILABLE CARB (g) PER SERVE	GL PER SERVE
Agave Nectar, premium, Sweet Cactus Farms	19	1 tsp, 5g	3	1
Brown rice syrup	98	10g	8	8
© Coles Simply Less Strawberry Fruit Spread	39	20g	6	2
© Coles Simply Less Raspberry Fruit Spread	39	20g	6	2
Coconut sugar	54	5g	5	3
Divine Date spread, Buderim Ginger	29	1 tbsp, 25g	16	5
Fruisana Fructose, pure	19	1 sachet, 10g	10	2
Ginger, sucrose free, Buderim Ginger	10	4 pieces, 20g	15	2
Golden syrup	63	2 tsp, 14g	10	6
Honey				
Blended	64	2 tsp, 14g	12	8
ironbark	48	2 tsp, 14g	12	6
red gum	53	2 tsp, 14g	12	6
Salvation Jane	64	2 tsp, 14g	12	8
stringybark	44	2 tsp, 14g	12	5
yapunya	52	2 tsp, 14g	12	6
yellowbox	35	2 tsp, 14g	12	4
Karo Dark Corn Syrup	90	30ml	22	20

★ little or no carbs ■ high in saturated fat ● untested/unknown © GI Symbol partner
Low GI = less than or equal to 55

SPREADS & SWEETENERS

FOOD	GI	SAMPLE SERVING	AVAILABLE CARB (g) PER SERVE	GI PER SERVE
Kraft Peanut Butter, smooth or crunchy	20	1 tbsp, 20g	4	1
Kraft Whipped Peanut Butter	19	1 tbsp, 15g	3	1
Maple-flavoured syrup, Cottees	68	1 tbsp, 20g	11	7
Maple syrup, pure	54	1 tbsp, 27g	18	10
Marmalade, ginger, Buderim Ginger	50	1 tbsp, 18g	13	7
Marmalade, orange	55	2 tbsp, 25g	16	9
Nutella, hazelnut spread, Ferrero	25	2 tsp, 10g	5	1
Strawberry jam, regular	51	1 tbsp, 25g	17	9
St Dalfour				
Black Cherry Jam	50	1 tbsp, 25g	13	6
Blackberry Jam	54	1 tbsp, 25g	13	7
Golden Peach Jam	50	1 tbsp, 25g	13	7
Gourmet Pear Jam	53	1 tbsp, 25g	13	7
Mirabelle Plum Jam	54	1 tbsp, 25g	13	7
Orange Marmalade	54	1 tbsp, 25g	14	8
Pineapple Mango Jam	55	1 tbsp, 25g	13	7
Raspberry & Pomegranate Jam	55	1 tbsp, 25g	14	8
Red Raspberry Jam	55	1 tbsp, 25g	14	8
Royal Fig Jam	51	1 tbsp, 25g	13	6

★ little or no carbs ■ high in saturated fat ● untested/unknown © GI Symbol partner
Low GI = less than or equal to 55

SPREADS & SWEETENERS

FOOD	GI	SAMPLE SERVING	AVAILABLE CARB (g) PER SERVE	GL PER SERVE
St Dalfour (continued)				
Strawberry Jam	52	1 tbsp, 25g	13	7
Thick Apricot Jam	54	1 tbsp, 25g	13	7
Wild Blueberry Jam	52	1 tbsp, 25g	13	7
Sugar	65	1 tsp, 5g	5	3
Treacle	68	3 tsp, 20g	13	9
Vinegar	★	1 tsp, 5ml	0	●

★ little or no carbs ■ high in saturated fat ● untested/unknown ⓒ GI Symbol partner
Low GI = less than or equal to 55

TAKEAWAY & PRE-PREPARED MEALS

FOOD	GI	SAMPLE SERVING	AVAILABLE CARB (g) PER SERVE	GL PER SERVE
Baked potato with baked beans	62	I serve, 140g	37	23
Battered fish, commercial	●	I serve, 100g	14	●
Burrito, corn tortilla, refried beans & tomato salsa	39	I serve, 100g	23	9
Cannelloni, spinach & ricotta, prepared convenience meal	15	I serve, 300g	54	8
Chicken nuggets, frozen, reheated in microwave 5 min	46■	6 nuggets, 100g	16	7
Chiko roll	●	I serve, 100g	26	●
Chips, takeaway	75	I serve, 100g	19	14
Crumbed calamari	●	I serve, 100g	16	●
Crumbed fish burger with cheese and tartar sauce	66■	I burger, 128g	30	20
Dim sim, commercial, deep fried	●	I serve, 100g	27	●
Dosai, served with chutney	55	I serve, 150g	39	21
Fajitas, chicken	42	I serve, 300g	42	18
Fish fingers	38	4 fingers, 100g	18	7

★ little or no carbs ■ high in saturated fat ● untested/unknown © GI Symbol partner
Low GI = less than or equal to 55

TAKEAWAY & PRE-PREPARED MEALS

FOOD	GI	SAMPLE SERVING	AVAILABLE CARB (g) PER SERVE	GL PER SERVE
French fries	75■	1 serve, 150g	29	22
Fried chicken e.g. KFC	●	1 serve, 100g	6	●
Fried fritter	69■	1 roll, 200g	35	24
Fried rice in Yangzhou-style	80	1 serve, 300g	69	55
Fried rice noodles with sliced beef	66	1 serve, 300g	60	40
Hamburger with beef patty, onion, mustard and tomato sauce	66	1 burger, 95g	25	17
Lasagne, beef, commercially made	47■	1 serve, 300g	35	16
Made For You Foods				
Beef Lasagne frozen meal	41	1 serve, 390g	55	22
Cottage Pie with Sweet Potato frozen meal	38	1 serve, 340g	30	12
Supreme Pizza frozen meal	53■	1 small pizza, 265g	46	24
Thai Green Chicken Curry frozen meal	50■	1 serve, 340g	33	17
Vegetable Lasagne frozen meal	45	1 serve, 380g	51	23

★ little or no carbs   ■ high in saturated fat   ● untested/unknown   ⓒ GI Symbol partner
Low GI = less than or equal to 55

TAKEAWAY & PRE-PREPARED MEALS

FOOD	GI	SAMPLE SERVING	AVAILABLE CARB (g) PER SERVE	GL PER SERVE
Meat pie	45■	1 regular, 175g	41	18
Moussaka, lamb, prepared convenience meal	35■	1 serve, 300g	27	9
Party pies, beef	45■	1 regular, 38g	10	5
Pasta sauce				
Latina Fresh varieties				
Bolognese sauce	24	½ tub, 212g	15	4
Creamy Sun dried tomato	19	½ tub, 212g	18	3
Italian tomato & garlic	40	½ tub, 212g	14	6
Mediterranean sauce	40	½ tub, 212g	10	4
Pizza Hut varieties				
Supreme, thin & crispy,	30■	1 slice, 71g	17	5
Super Supreme, pan	36■	1 slice, 94	23	8
Veggie Supreme, thin & crispy	49■	1 slice, 63g	16	8
Pork Bun, Asian, commercial	69	1 bun, 60g	25	17
Pork Puff, Asian, BBQ pork, commercial	55■	1 portion, 54g	17	9
Potato scallop	●	1 serve, 100g	27	●

★ little or no carbs　■ high in saturated fat　● untested/unknown　© GI Symbol partner
Low GI = less than or equal to 55

TAKEAWAY & PRE-PREPARED MEALS

FOOD	GI	SAMPLE SERVING	AVAILABLE CARB (g) PER SERVE	GL PER SERVE
Sausages and mash, prepared, convenience meal	61■	I serve, 500g	67	41
Shepherd's pie	66	I serve, 500g	74	49
Singapore fried vermicelli noodles	54■	I serve, 300g	45	24
Soups				
Barley & vegetable	41	I cup, 250ml	28	11
Campbell's Country Ladle Chicken & vegetable with wholegrain pasta	43	½ can, 250ml	9	4
Minestrone, traditional	39	I can, 290ml	18	7
Carrot, canned	35	I cup, 250ml	13	5
Chicken & mushroom	58	I cup, 250ml	18	10
Clear consommé, chicken or vegetable	★	I cup, 205ml	0	●
Green pea, canned	66	I cup, 250ml	41	27
Lentil, canned	44	I cup, 250ml	21	9
Pumpkin, creamy, Heinz Very Special	76	I cup, 290ml	29	22

★ little or no carbs   ■ high in saturated fat   ● untested/unknown   © GI Symbol partner
Low GI = less than or equal to 55

TAKEAWAY & PRE-PREPARED MEALS

FOOD	GI	SAMPLE SERVING	AVAILABLE CARB (g) PER SERVE	GL PER SERVE
Spicy Thai instant soup, low fat	56	1 cup, 250ml	31	17
Split pea, canned	60	1 cup, 250ml	27	16
Tomato, canned	45	1 cup, 250ml	17	8
Vegetable	60	1 cup, 250ml	18	11
Spring Roll	50■	1 roll, 80g	18	9
Spaghetti Bolognaise	52	1 serve, 360g	48	25
Steak, mashed potato & mixed vegetables, homemade	66	1 serve, 360g	53	35
Steamed Vermicelli roll	90	1 roll, 190g	40	36
Steamed Glutinous Rice roll	89	1 roll, 94g	43	39
Sticky Rice in Lotus Leaf	83	1 serve, 300g	89	74
Sushi, tofu and pickled radish nori roll with brown rice, Keepin it Fresh	45	1 roll, 200g	42	19
Sushi, salmon	48	2 med pieces, 100g	14	7

★ little or no carbs ■ high in saturated fat ● untested/unknown © GI Symbol partner
Low GI = less than or equal to 55

185

TAKEAWAY & PRE-PREPARED MEALS

FOOD	GI	SAMPLE SERVING	AVAILABLE CARB (g) PER SERVE	GL PER SERVE
Taco shells, cornmeal-based, baked	68	2 regular, 26g	14	10
Vine leaves, stuffed with rice & lamb, served with tomato sauce	30	1 serve, 100g	15	5

★ little or no carbs ■ high in saturated fat ● untested/unknown ⓖ GI Symbol partner
Low GI = less than or equal to 55

VEGETABLES

FOOD	GI	SAMPLE SERVING	AVAILABLE CARB (g) PER SERVE	GL PER SERVE
Starchy vegetables				
Beetroot, fresh, boiled	●	I whole, 82g	7	●
Beetroot, canned	64	4 slices, 32g	3	2
Carrot	39	I medium, 60g	3	I
Carrot juice	43	I cup, 250ml	14	6
Cassava, peeled, diced, boiled	46	I cup, 140g	42	19
Corn on cob	48	I medium, 80g	16	8
Corn, loose kernels	48	½ cup, 90g	17	8
Corn, canned	46	½ cup, 88g	16	7
Corn, creamed, canned	●	⅓ can, 86g	14	●
French fries	75■	I serve, 150g	29	22
Mixed vegetables, frozen e.g., peas, carrot, swede, beans, sweet corn	●	½ cup	II	●
Parsnip, boiled	52	I cup, 100g	10	5
Parsnip, baked	●	100g	12	●
Peas, green, fresh or frozen, boiled	51	½ cup, 80g	6	3

★ little or no carbs ■ high in saturated fat ● untested/unknown ⓒ GI Symbol partner
Low GI = less than or equal to 55

VEGETABLES

FOOD	GI	SAMPLE SERVING	AVAILABLE CARB (g) PER SERVE	GL PER SERVE
Starchy vegetables (continued)				
Peas, canned	●	100g	9	●
Potato, baked, peeled, without oil	●	2 med chunks, 100g	20	●
Potato, baked, jacket, in foil, without oil	●	1 large, 200g	28	●
ⓖ Potato, Baby Carisma, unpeeled, boiled 8 min (or until al dente), Coles	55	22g	12	6
ⓖ Potato, Carisma, unpeeled, boiled 8 min (or until al dente), Coles	55	1 medium, 125g	16	9
Potato chips, frozen, oven heat	●	15–20 chips, 100g	45	●
Potato, Desiree, peeled, boiled 35 min	101	1 medium, 150g	17	17
Potato, French fries	75■	1 serve, 150g	29	22
Potato Gems	●	12 gems	31	●
Potato, Hash Browns, Birds Eye	56	1 hash brown, 62g	11	6
Potato, mashed, instant, Edgell	86	¼ pkt, 150g	20	17

★ little or no carbs ■ high in saturated fat ● untested/unknown ⓖ GI Symbol partner
Low GI = less than or equal to 55

VEGETABLES

FOOD	GI	SAMPLE SERVING	AVAILABLE CARB (g) PER SERVE	GL PER SERVE
Starchy vegetables (continued)				
Potato, mashed potato, with butter and milk	●	½ cup, 100g	11	●
Potato, Nadine				
baked	54	150g	20	11
boiled	49	150g	20	10
microwave	57	150g	20	11
Potato, new	78	2 small, 140g	18	14
Potato, new, canned, microwaved	65	3–4 small, 120g	17	11
Potato, Nicola, unpeeled, boiled whole 15 min	58	3 small, 150g	16	9
Potato, Pontiac, peeled, boiled 15 min, mashed	91	½ cup, 150g	20	18
Potato Pontiac, peeled, boiled whole 30–35 min	72	1 medium, 150g	18	13
Potato Pontiac, peeled, microwaved 7 min	79	1 medium, 150g	18	14
Potato, Sebago, peeled, boiled 35 min	87	1 medium, 150g	17	15

★ little or no carbs ■ high in saturated fat ● untested/unknown ⓒ GI Symbol partner
Low GI = less than or equal to 55

VEGETABLES

FOOD	GI	SAMPLE SERVING	AVAILABLE CARB (g) PER SERVE	GL PER SERVE
Starchy vegetables (continued)				
Potato, wedges, with skin, frozen, oven heat	●	2 large, 50g	44	●
Pumpkin, baked	●	1 cup, 100g	8	●
Pumpkin, boiled	66	1 cup, 100g	7	5
Pumpkin, butternut, boiled	51	1 cup, 100g	8	4
Swede, diced	72	1 cup, 170g	7	5
Sweet potato, orange, peeled, cut into pieces, boiled 8 min	61	100g	15	9
Sweet potato, purple skin white flesh, peeled, cut into pieces, boiled 8 min	75	1 cup, 150g	21	16
Tapioca, boiled	93	1 cup, 250g	18	17
Tapioca, pudding, creamed, homemade	81	1 cup	35	28
Taro	54	½ cup, 100g	25	14
Yam, peeled, boiled	54	1 cup, 100g	25	14

★ little or no carbs ■ high in saturated fat ● untested/unknown ©️ GI Symbol partner
Low GI = less than or equal to 55

VEGETABLES

FOOD	GI	SAMPLE SERVING	AVAILABLE CARB (g) PER SERVE	GL PER SERVE
Green/salad vegetables				
Alfalfa sprouts	★	6g	0	●
Artichokes, globe, fresh or canned in brine	★	80g	0	●
Artichoke, Jerusalem	●	3 medium, 145g	13	●
Asparagus	★	100g	0	●
Bean sprouts, raw	★	14g	0	●
Bok choy	★	100g	0	●
Broad beans, fresh, raw	●	½ cup, 55g	1	●
Broad beans, frozen, reheated	63	½ cup, 75g	8	5
Broccoli	★	60g	0	●
Brussels sprouts	★	100g	0	●
Cabbage	★	70g	0	●
Capsicum	★	80g	0	●
Cauliflower	★	60g	0	●
Celery	★	40g	0	●
Chillies, fresh or dried	★	20g	0	●

★ little or no carbs ■ high in saturated fat ● untested/unknown ⓒ GI Symbol partner
Low GI = less than or equal to 55

VEGETABLES

FOOD	GI	SAMPLE SERVING	AVAILABLE CARB (g) PER SERVE	GL PER SERVE
Green/salad vegetables (continued)				
Chives, fresh	★	4g	0	●
Cucumber	★	45g	0	●
Eggplant	★	100g	0	●
Endive	★	30g	0	●
Fennel	★	90g	0	●
Garlic	★	5g	0	●
Ginger	★	10g	0	●
Herbs, fresh or dried	★	2g	0	●
Leeks	★	80g	0	●
Lettuce	★	50g	0	●
Mushrooms	★	35g	0	●
Okra	★	80g	0	●
Onions, raw, peeled	★	30g	0	●
Onions, stir-fried without extra oil	★	100g	8	●
Radishes	★	15g	0	●

★ little or no carbs   ■ high in saturated fat   ● untested/unknown   ⓖ GI Symbol partner
Low GI = less than or equal to 55

VEGETABLES

FOOD	GI	SAMPLE SERVING	AVAILABLE CARB (g) PER SERVE	GL PER SERVE
Green/salad vegetables (continued)				
Rocket	★	30g	0	●
Shallots	★	10g	0	●
Silverbeet	★	35g	0	●
Snowpea sprouts	★	15g	0	●
Spinach	★	75g	0	●
Spring onions	★	15g	0	●
Squash, yellow	★	70g	0	●
Tomato	★	150g	0	●
Turnip	★	120g	0	●
Watercress	★	8g	0	●
Zucchini	★	100g	0	●

★ little or no carbs ■ high in saturated fat ● untested/unknown Ⓖ GI Symbol partner
Low GI = less than or equal to 55

WEIGHT MANAGEMENT PRODUCTS

FOOD	GI	SAMPLE SERVING	AVAILABLE CARB (g) PER SERVE	GL PER SERVE
Achievit VLED				
Shake (Chocolate, Vanilla, Strawberry and Caffe Latte flavours)	22	52g powder	17–18	4
Soup (Creamy Chicken or Cream of Tomato and Veg)	20	50g powder	17	3
Blackmores				
Superfruit Smoothie Meal Replacement				
Creamy Vanilla	17	45g powder	18	3
Dark Chocolate & Blackcurrant	21	45g powder	17	4
Mixed Berries	23	45g powder	18	4
Herbalife				
Formula 1 Nutritional Shake Mix				
French Vanilla	20	28g powder + 300ml water	15	3
Dutch Chocolate	19	28g powder + 300ml water	1	3
Berry	21	28g powder + 300ml water	15	3
Cookies 'n' Cream	15	28g powder + 300ml water	15	3

★ little or no carbs   ■ high in saturated fat   ● untested/unknown   ☺ GI Symbol partner
Low GI = less than or equal to 55

WEIGHT MANAGEMENT PRODUCTS

FOOD	GI	SAMPLE SERVING	AVAILABLE CARB (g) PER SERVE	GL PER SERVE
IsoWhey Complete				
Double Chocolate meal replacement beverage	23	35g + 200ml water	6	1
French Vanilla meal replacement beverage	30	32g + 200ml water	8	1
Strawberries & Cream meal replacement beverage	30	32g + 200ml water	8	1
© Nutrimeal Chocolate Whey meal replacement drink, prepared with water	25	1 cup, 250ml	25	7
© Nutrimeal Free Vanilla, Usana	49	290ml with water	18	9
© Nutrimeal Dutch Chocolate	25	60g powder	24	6
© Nutrimeal French Vanilla	25	60g powder	24	6
© Nutrimeal Strawberry	25	60g powder	24	6
Optifast VLCD varieties				
© Banana Shake	24	54g powder	23	6
© Caramel Shake	34	54g powder	23	8
© Chocolate Shake	31	54g powder	23	7
© Coffee Shake	31	54g powder	23	7
© Strawberry Shake	27	54g powder	23	6
© Vanilla Shake	27	54g powder	23	6
© Berry Crunch Bar	25	1 bar 60g	21	5
© Cappuccino Flavour Bar	29	1 bar 60g	20	6
© Chocolate Bar	20	1 bar 70g	13	3

★ little or no carbs ■ high in saturated fat ● untested/unknown © GI Symbol partner
Low GI = less than or equal to 55

WEIGHT MANAGEMENT PRODUCTS

FOOD	GI	SAMPLE SERVING	AVAILABLE CARB (g) PER SERVE	GL PER SERVE
☺ Chicken Flavour Soup	31	48g powder	17	5
☺ Tomato Soup	25	54g powder	22	6
☺ Vegetable Soup	24	54g powder	13	3
☺ Chocolate Dessert	27	46g powder	17	5
☺ Lemon Creme Flavour Dessert	27	46g powder	17	5
Proform				
Neutral Formulated Meal Replacement	42	60g powder	34	14
Vanilla Formulated Meal Replacement	45	60g powder	37	17
Chocolate Formulated Meal Replacement	43	60g powder	37	16
Reduce XS Chocolate Deluxe formulated meal replacement powder, prepared with water	10	1 cup, 250ml	8	1
Slim Fast French Vanilla ready-to-drink shake	37	1 can, 325ml	35	13

★ little or no carbs ■ high in saturated fat ● untested/unknown ☺ GI Symbol partner
Low GI = less than or equal to 55

WEIGHT MANAGEMENT PRODUCTS

FOOD	GI	SAMPLE SERVING	AVAILABLE CARB (g) PER SERVE	GL PER SERVE
Tony Ferguson				
Apricot Munch Bar	51	1 bar, 60g	26	13
Berry Munch Bar	43	1 bar, 60g	28	12
Crème of Chicken Soup	26	58g powder	31	8
Meal Replacement Shake, all flavours, prepared with water	22	1 cup, 250ml	28	6
Mixed Berry Muesli, prepared with water	32	1 sachet, 56g	28	9
Mixed Nut Snack Bar	37	1 bar, 30g	13	5
Raspberry & Cranberry, prepared with water	32	1 sachet, 56g	28	9
Ready to Drink Shakes (Chocolate, Espresso flavours)	20	375 ml	29–31	6
Roast Pumpkin Soup	27	58g powder	29	8
Shakes (Chocolate, Espresso, Café Latte flavours)	22	53g powder	29–30	6
Sweet Chilli & Sour Cream, Munch Bar	35	1 bar, 60g	21	7

★ little or no carbs ■ high in saturated fat ● untested/unknown ⓒ GI Symbol partner
Low GI = less than or equal to 55

Visit the Glycemic Index Foundation's website www.gisymbol.com for information and the latest news on the Glycemic Index of foods.

You will find:

- *GI News*, the free newsletter featuring the latest research on the glycemic index, carbohydrates, diet and diabetes, along with other hot nutrition topics

- The benefits of consuming low GI foods for diabetes, weight management and sustained energy

- Glycemic Load explained

- Simple swap tool

- Recipes

- Top tips to go low GI

- Fact sheets, toolkits and more

The GI Symbol: Making healthier low GI choices easy.

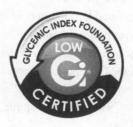

www.glycemicindex.com

Search our database for the latest foods tested at the home of the Glycemic Index and discover the answers to the 20 most frequently asked questions about the glycemic index.

- What is the difference between glycemic index (GI) and glycemic load (GL)?
- Should I use GI or GL and does it really matter?
- Do I need to eat only low GI foods at every meal to see a benefit?
- Why do many high-fibre foods still have a high GI value?
- Can I download or can you email me a full list of all GI food values?
- Does the GI increase with serving size? If I eat twice as much, does the GI double?
- If testing continued long enough, wouldn't you expect the areas under the curve to become equal, even for very high and very low GI foods?
- Why doesn't the GI of beef, chicken, fish, tofu, eggs, nuts, seeds, avocados, many fruits (including berries) and vegetables, wine, beer and spirits appear on the GI database?

- Some vegetables appear to have a high GI. Does this mean a person with diabetes should avoid eating them?
- Can you tell me the GI of alcoholic beverages (beer, wine and spirits)?
- Why does some variability occur in the GI for the same food types?
- Why does pasta have a low GI?
- Most breads and potatoes have a high GI. Does this mean I should never eat them?
- What about flour? If I make my own bread (or dumplings, pancakes, muffins etc) which flours, if any, are low GI? What about sprouted grain breads?
- Some high fat foods have a low GI. Doesn't this give a falsely favourable impression of that food?
- Why not just adopt a low carbohydrate diet (like the Atkins diet) to keep my blood glucose levels and weight down?
- Is there a GI Plan for nursing mothers?
- How relevant is the GI for athletes?
- I have recently been diagnosed with coeliac disease (gluten sensitivity). It's extremely hard to find both low GI and wheat-free foods. Any suggestions?
- Is a low GI diet suitable for vegetarians?

Your GI Favourites – Low GI

Your GI Favourites – Higher GI

Your GI Favourites – Low GI

Your GI Favourites – Higher GI

Food index

Where to go for further help

For further information on GI
www.glycemicindex.com
This is the University of Sydney's glycemic index website where you can learn about GI and access the GI database which includes the most up-to-date listing of the GI of foods that have been published in international scientific journals.

www.gisymbol.com
The Glycemic Index (GI) Symbol Program is a food labelling program with strict nutritional criteria that aims to help people make informed food choices. The site includes a complete listing of foods carrying the GI symbol and information on the benefits of eating low GI foods.

www.gisymbol.com/ginews
GI News is the University of Sydney Human Nutrition Unit's official glycemic index monthly newletter. Subscribing is free.

For information on:

Food labelling and food additives
Food Standards Australia New Zealand (FSANZ)
www.foodstandards.gov.au

Finding a dietitian
Dietitians Association of Australia (DAA)
www.daa.asn.au

Dietitians New Zealand
www.dietitians.org.nz

Diabetes Australia
www.diabetesaustralia.com.au

Diabetes New Zealand
www.diabetes.org.nz

JDRF (Australia)
www.jdrf.org.au

Heart health
Heart Foundation of Australia
www.heartfoundation.org.au

Heart Foundation of New Zealand
www.heartfoundation.org.nz

Te Hotu Manawa Maori
This is a national health promotion organisation with the specific aim of reducing the likelihood of heart-related illness and death amongst Maori. They undertake training courses for Maori in nutrition and physical activity.
www.tehotumanawa.org.nz

Coeliac Disease
Coeliac Australia
www.coeliac.org.au

Coeliac New Zealand
www.coeliac.org.nz

The following brands that appear in this shopping guide are trademarks™ or registered trademarks®:

Bill's Organic Bread, Blackmores, Blu Gourmet Pearl Couscous, Buderim Ginger, Carman's, Defiance, Golden Circle, Harrod Foods, Isostar, IsoWhey Complete, Kavli, Keepin it Fresh, Lucozade, Made For You, Monster Muesli, Mr Kipling, Nature First Organic, Naturis Organic Breads, Nudie, Orgran, Pav's Bakery, Pink Lady, Pom Wonderful, Proform, ProteinFX, Pringles, ReduceXS, St. Dalfour, Sweetaddin, Tony Ferguson Weightloss Program, Yakult, Yummiees, Wild About Fruit.

The following brands that appear in this guide are trademarks™ or registered trademarks® of their respective companies:

Abbott Laboratories: Ensure, Jevity.
ALDI Foods Pty Ltd: Dairy Dream.
Arnott's Biscuits Australia: Breton, Cruskits, Full o' Fruit, Ginger Nut, Jatz, Jatz 97% fat free, Malt-O-Milk, Marie, Milk Arrowroot, Morning Coffee, Salada, Sao, Shapes, Shredded Wheatmeal, Snack Right, Spicy Fruit Roll, Thin Captain, Vita-Weat.
Asahi Group Holdings, Ltd: Schweppes, Solo.
Aussie Bodies Pty. Ltd., Australia: Healtheries, Trim Low-GI Protein Snacks.
Bakers Delight Holdings Limited: Bakers Delight, Fit2Go Bars.
Bathox Australia Pty Ltd: Sugarless.
Campbell's Soups Australia: Campbell's, Campbell's Country Ladle.
Capitol Chilled Foods Pty Ltd, ACT, Australia: Chris' Traditional.
Capital Foods Pty Ltd, Australia: Casa Fiesta.
Celanese Corporation: Sunnett.
Coca-Cola Company, Atlanta, GA, USA: Coca-Cola, Fanta.
Coles Supermarkets Australia Pty Ltd: Coles.
CSR: LoGiCane.
Danisco USA Inc: Aclame, Fruisana.
Ferrero: Nutella.
Fonterra Brands Pty Ltd: Tamar Valley.
Freedom Foods: Australia's Own, Gluten-Free Muesli, FreeOats Crunchola, Hi-Lite Breakfast Bar, Omega Bar, Quick Oats Porridge, Superberry Breakfast Bar, Yeast-free Muesli.
George Weston Foods Limited: Bürgen, Golden, Noble Rise, Tip Top, Tip Top 9-Grain, Tip Top Sunblest.
General Mills Ltd: Betty Crocker, Latina Fresh.
GlaxoSmithKline group of companies: Ribena, Goodness Superfoods Digestive 1st, Heart 1st, Protein 1st.
Golden Hearth, a division of Gold Coast Bakeries: Organic Heavy Wholegrain.
Goodman Fielder: Buttercup, Country Life, Molenberg, Paradise, Wonder White.
Green's General Foods Pty Ltd: Green's, Lowan Whole Foods, Poppin.
Griffin's Food Limited, New Zealand: Fruitli Golden Fruit, Maltmeal Wafer.

Gruma Corporation, USA: Mission Foods.
H.J. Heinz Company Australia Ltd's: Cottee's, Heinz.
Hermanbrot Pty Ltd: Herman Brot.
Hermes Sweeteners Ltd: Hermesetas.
Inova Pharmaceuticals: Glucodin.
Jalna Dairy Foods, VIC, Australia: Jalna.
Johnson & Johnson: Splenda.
Kellogg's, a division of Kellogg (Aust) Pty Ltd: All-Bran, Be Natural, Corn
    Flakes, Crispix, Crunchy Nut Clusters, Crunchy Nut Corn Flakes, Froot
    Loops, Frosties, Fruit & Nut Medley, Guardian, Just Right, Mini-Wheats,
    Nutri-Grain, Rice Bubbles, Special K, Special K Advantage, Sultana Bran,
    Sultana Bran Crunch.
Kraft Foods Inc.: belVita Breakfast, Kraft.
Lighthouse Asset Management Pty Ltd: Carman's
Lindt & Sprüngli: Lindt Lindor
Lion Nathan National Foods: Tooheys.
Mars Confectionery: Dove, M&M's, Mars Bar, Skittles, Snickers, Twix,
    Uncle Ben's.
Mersiant, USA: Equal, Equal Spoonful
The Mitolo Group: Carisma potatoes
Lighthouse Asset Management Pty Ltd: Carman's
Morning Sun, a division of Cereal Partners Worldwide, a division of Nestlé:
    Morning Sun Apricot & Almond Muesli, Fruit-free Nuts & Seeds Muesli,
    Peach & Pecan Muesli.
National Foods: Berri, Big M, Daily Juice Co., Dairy Farmers, Farmer's Best,
    Fruche, Masters, Pura, Quelch, Shape, Yogo, Yoplait, Yoplait Formé,
    Yoplait Go Gurt, Yoplait Le Rice.
Naturex, France: Talin.
Nutrasweet Property Holding Inc, USA: Nutrasweet.
Ocean Spray International, Inc.: Ocean Spray.
Parmalat Australia Ltd (formerly Pauls Limited): Vaalia, Paul's, Rush.
Paradise Foods Australia: Vive Lites, Vive Wellbeing.
PR Nutrition, San Diego, CA, USA: Ironman PR Bar.
Profile Foods Ltd, NZ: Mother Earth.
Real Foods Pty Ltd: Corn Thins.
Reckitt Benkiser: Sugarine, Sweetex
Regal Cream Products Pty Ltd: Bulla.
Rice Growers Limited: SunRice, SunGold, Sunbrown Quick, Doongara
    CleverRice, SunRice.
Riviana Foods: Mahatma.
San Diego Tortilla Factory Pty Ltd: Diego's
Sara Lee Corporation: Sara Lee.
Sanitarium Health Foods, Australia: Bran Flakes, Fibre Life, Granola
    Clusters, Hi-Bran Weet-Bix, Honey Weets, Light 'n' Tasty, Puffed Wheat,
    Sanitarium, Skippy Cornflakes, So Good, Up&Go, Up&Go Vive, Weet-Bix.
Sanofi ANZ: Sugarella.
Simplot Australia subsidiary of the J R Simplot Company: Birds Eye, Edgell.
Smith's Snackfood Company: Burger Rings, Grain Waves, Parker's Pretzels,
    Smith's, Twisties.

Société des Produits Nestlé S.A.: Life Savers, Maggi, Milky Bar, Milky Way, Milo, Nesquik, Optifast VLCD, Peter's, Sustagen, Uncle Tobys, Uncle Tobys Bran Plus, Uncle Tobys Cheerios, Uncle Tobys Farmer's Pick, Uncle Tobys Fruit Roll-Ups, Uncle Tobys Healthwise for Heart Wellbeing, Uncle Tobys O&G, Uncle Tobys Oatbrits, Uncle Tobys Original Swiss Style Muesli, Uncle Tobys Quick Oats, Uncle Tobys Vita Brits, Uncle Tobys Weeties.

SPC Ardmona Operations Limited (SPCA): SPC.

STM Ltd: Chiko.

Stokely-Van Camp Inc, USA: Gatorade.

Sunbeam Foods, Vic: Sunbeam.

Susan Day Cakes, Vic, Aust: Big Sister Foods.

Unilever Australiasia: Continental, Slim Fast.

Usana Inc: Usana Nutrimeal.

Valeant Pharmaceuticals International Inc: Achievit

Vetta pasta: Vetta.

Vitasoy Australia Products: Vitasoy.

Vitasoy International Holdings Ltd: Vita Go.

Vogel's, a division of Specialty Cereals: Grain Clusters, Muesli Cluster Spice, Muesli Fruit & Nut, Ultra-Bran.

Weight Watchers, a division of HJ Heinz Australia: Butternut Cookies, Fruit Slice, Triple Chocolate Cookies.

Wendy's Supa Sundaes Pty Ltd, Australia: Wendy's, Chocollo.

Wilson Foods Ltd, NZ: Sucaryl.

Woolworths Limited: Naytura, Woolworth's Select.

Yum! Brands: KFC, Pizza Hut.